Controlled Release Nitroglycerin in Buccal and Oral Form

Advances in Pharmacotherapy

Vol. 1

Series Editors
G. Stille, Berlin; *W. Wagner,* Dortmund, and
W.M. Herrmann, Berlin

KARGER
Basel · München · Paris · London · New York · Tokyo · Sydney

3rd Workshop in Kronberg, Kronberg/Taunus, September 9–10, 1981

Controlled Release Nitroglycerin in Buccal and Oral Form

Volume Editors
W.-D. Bussmann, Frankfurt a.M.; *R.-R. Dries,* Kiel, and
W. Wagner, Dortmund

81 figures, 2 colour plates, and 52 tables, 1982

KARGER
Basel · München · Paris · London · New York · Tokyo · Sydney

Translation into English of the contributions Windorfer, Hummerich et al., Langbehn et al., Kaiser et al., Ohlmeier et al., Mertens et al., Prager, Lehmann et al., Konrads et al., Schneider et al., and of the discussions by *Angelika Beisel,* MD, and *Andrew Jenkins,* BA.

National Library of Medicine, Cataloging in Publication
Controlled release nitroglycerin in buccal and oral form
3rd workshop in Kronberg, Kronberg/Taunus, September 9–10, 1981
Volume editors, W.-D. Bussmann, R.-R. Dries, and W. Wagner. – Basel; New York: Karger, 1982.
(Advances in pharmacotherapy; v.1)
1. Glyceryl Trinitrate – administration and dosage – congresses 2. Glyceryl Trinitrate – pharmacodynamics – congresses I. Bussmann, W.-D. II. Dries, R.-R. III. Wagner, W. (Wolfgang) IV. Series
W1 AD78N v.1 [QV 156 C764 1981]
ISBN 3–8055–3507–4

Drug Dosage

The authors and publisher have exerted every effort to ensure that drug selection and dosage set forth in this text are in accord with current recommendations and practice at the time of publication. However, in view of ongoing research, changes in government regulations, and the constant flow of information relating to drug therapy and drug reactions, the reader is urged to check the package insert for each drug for any change in indications and dosage and for added warnings and precautions. This is particularly important when the recommended agent is a new and/or infrequently employed drug.

Printed in Switzerland by Thür AG Offsetdruck, Pratteln
ISBN 3–8055–3507–4

Contents

Preface VIII
Acknowledgements XI

Bussmann, W.-D. (Frankfurt a.M.): Introduction 1

Overview: Indications for Nitroglycerin

Abrams, J. (Albuquerque, N. Mex.): Nitroglycerin and Long-Acting Nitrates: A Contemporary Perspective 4

The Synchron Controlled Release System

Davis, S.S.; Daly, P.B.; Kennerley, J.W.; Frier, M.; Hardy, J.G.; Wilson, C.G. (Nottingham): Design and Evaluation of Sustained Release Formulations for Oral and Buccal Administration 17

Pharmacology of Buccal and Oral Nitroglycerin

Fung, H.-L. (Buffalo, N.Y.): Factors Affecting the Determination and Interpretation of Nitroglycerin Pharmacokinetics 26
Erb, R.J. (West Lafayette, Ind.): Bioavailability of Controlled Release Buccal and Oral Nitroglycerin by Digital Plethysmography 35
Windorfer, A. (Freiburg i.Br.): Nitroglycerin Blood Level after Buccal and Oral Application of Synchron Nitroglycerin 44

Special Mechanism of Action

Hummerich, W.; Konrads, A.; Wambach, G.; Meurer, K.A.; Dries, R.-R.; Langbehn, A.-F. (Köln/Lünen/Bad Segeberg): Effects of Nitroglycerin on Vasopressin Release and the Renin-Angiotensin-Aldosterone System in Man 49

Niehues, B.; Thoma, R. (Köln): Hemodynamics and Lung Function in Patients with Chronic Obstructive Lung Disease following Administration of Nitroglycerin and Aminophylline 57

Clinical Results with Buccal Nitroglycerin

Bussmann, W.-D.; Kromm, W.; Reifart, N.; Fung, H.-L. (Frankfurt a.M./Buffalo, N.Y.): Acute Hemodynamic and Pharmacokinetic Effects of Buccal Nitroglycerin 64

Langbehn, A.-F.; Beurich, H.W.; Leupold, H.; Hoffmann, R.; Sheikhzaden, A.; Lohaus, R. (Bad Segeberg/Lünen): Effect of Buccal Synchron Nitroglycerin on Pulmonary Artery Pressure at Rest and during Exercise. A Comparison with Sublingual Nitroglycerin in Patients with Coronary Artery Disease 73

Kaiser, D.; Tegen, W.; Langbehn, A.-F.; Hoppe, M. (Bad Segeberg): Acute Effect of Buccal Synchron Nitroglycerin on Pacer-Induced Angina pectoris and Left Ventricular Enddiastolic Pressure 98

Ohlmeier, H.; Mertens, H.M.; Mannebach, H.; Gleichmann, U. (Bad Oeynhausen): Effect of Buccally Administered Synchron Nitroglycerin on Pulmonary Artery Pressure. A Comparison with Sublingually Administered Nitroglycerin in Patients with Coronary Heart Disease 101

Mertens, H.M.; Ohlmeier, H.; Mannebach, H.; Gleichmann, U. (Bad Oeynhausen): Changes in Left Ventricular Hemodynamics under Buccal Synchron Nitroglycerin. A Noninvasive Study Using Systolic Time Intervals 116

Prager, G.; Wagner, W. (Regensburg/Dortmund): Cold-Induced Angina pectoris. Acute Prophylaxis and Long-Term Protection by Controlled-Release Buccal Nitroglycerin 123

Prager, G. (Regensburg): Buccal Synchron Nitroglycerin in Acute Treatment of Angina pectoris Attacks. A Comparison with Sublingually Administered Nitroglycerin in Patients with Stable Coronary Artery Disease 137

Reichek, N.; Priest, C.; Kienzle, M.; Kleaveland, J.P.; Bolton, S.; St. John Sutton, M. (Philadelphia, Pa.): Angina Prophylaxis with Buccal Synchron Nitroglycerin: A Rapid Onset Long-Acting Nitrate 143

Reichek, N.; Priest, Ch.J.; St. John Sutton, M. (Philadelphia, Pa.): Long-Term Buccal Administration of Synchron Nitroglycerin 155

Lichstein, E.; Greengart, A.; Bolton, S.; Hollander, G.; Sanders, M. (New York, N.Y.): Efficacy of Buccal Synchron Nitroglycerin in Patients with Angina pectoris 166

Lichstein, E.; Greengart, A.; Hollander, G.; Sanders, M.; Cohen, G. (Brooklyn, N.Y.): Open Study of Safety and Tolerability of Nitroglycerin Buccal Controlled Release Tablet 174

Clinical Results with Oral Nitroglycerin

Lehmann, H.-U.; Witt, E.; Traue, P.; Hochrein, H. (Berlin): Hemodynamic Effects of Oral Synchron Nitroglycerin in Comparison to Slow-Release Isosorbide Dinitrate 184

Konrads, A.; Hummerich, W.; Strödter, H.; Dries, R.-R. (Köln/Lünen): Efficacy and Dosage of Oral Synchron Nitroglycerin in Patients with Coronary Heart Disease 194

Schneider, W.; Stahl, B.; Kaltenbach, M.; Bussmann, W.-D. (Frankfurt a.M.): Dose-Response Relationship of Oral Nitroglycerin in the Treatment of Coronary Heart Disease 204

Bussmann, W.-D. (Frankfurt a.M.): Summary 210

Subject Index 215

Preface

When the decision is taken to initiate a book series on 'Advances in Pharmacotherapy' at the beginning of the eighties in the 20th century, a number of questions arises:

What does advancement actually mean? Is progress in pharmacotherapy at all possible? Or has the traditional scientific approach to pharmaceutical research, the world-wide basis of which in our days predominantly lies in the principle of molecular variation, reached its culminating point or has it even gone beyond?

It is certain that we are in a process of permanent development and revolution. History is synonymous with change, and this is to a large extent also true for medicine and pharmacology. The medical historian *H. Schipperges* from Heidelberg makes this clear in his essay 'Structure and Change of Materia Medica': 'In pharmacology precisely, the old and the new cannot be clearly separated; the changeable and the unchangeable are closely related to each other; destruction and preservation complete each other individually as do annihilation and creation in its entirety. Only in this way is structure subject to change.'

The handling of the term 'advancement' requires modesty: (1) Statements are valid only within the respective scientific rationale and are based on model conceptions. (2) Within a changing scope also a critical position finding should be accepted as progress. This means it is also considered to be a progress if the therapeutic efficacy of a known drug can, for the first time, be established beyond any doubts or when, for the first time, plausible arguments have been collected leading to the conclusion that a recognized principle of action has to be considered obsolete. (3) Progress can also be found in what initially has been payed little attention to; new principles are not necessarily represented by means of traditional models.

The vested old and the new as well are milestones along the road towards progress. The new only gains in profile when measured by standards of the old. Subsequent definitions and confirmations of mechanisms of action can represent as much an advancement as the creating of new forms of application or new therapeutic systems. Advances are also a lower incidence of side effects with equal therapeutic efficacy, an improved therapeutic profile of action for equal indications, a lower dosage or new fields of application of already known drugs. Finally, the optimizing and extending of clinical-pharmacological methodology can entail advances in pharmacotherapy: echocardiography as non-invasive method for evaluating positive and negative inotropic substances, pharmaco-electroencephalography for an early classification of effects caused by psychotropic drugs or for detecting undesirable central nervous effects, the body plethysmography for objectifying bronchial obstruction, or the extending of 'therapeutic research' to the concept of 'therapeutic evaluation' by including scientific parameters related to social life, behavior and economics may serve as examples for this.

He who is in favor of progress ought to remain modest. Even a small step, an insignificant molecular modification may be part of the great development. He who wants to launch out must not ignore the steps. It was only one single chlorine atom which lead from Promazine to the first antipsychotic drug Chlorpromazine; a few methyl groups only, more or less, are the hormonal determinant of our sex characteristics. Trivial molecular manipulations in the opinion of critics of pharmacological research.

But progress, after all, means opening the conscience to new dimensions, thus not only the empirical but also the ontal. It is not only that discoveries made in the laboratories of industry and university often bear the 'stigma of fatigue' which marks the road to progress with sweat and tears, but also the sometimes erratic perception of connections.

Patterns of thought are tools of everyday life, the brilliant idea remains a rare event. The standard for every progress in pharmacotherapy is the patient. His diseases as well as symptoms standing for a disease require treatment. Only in the hands of the physician is a drug of direct value. A conscientious diagnosis and a careful selection of the drug finally determine the success.

A book series on 'Advances in Pharmacotherapy' is, therefore, mainly intended for the physician. The editors of the series 'Advances in Pharmacotherapy' will strive to consider as many aspects as possible; in order to accomplish this task they wish to identify themselves with two principles: critical rationalism as the scientific understanding of clinical pharmacology and modesty in the interpretation of the term advancement, as is appropriate to a discipline that is undergoing a continuous change.

Berlin and Dortmund, November 1981

Günther Stille
Wolfgang Wagner
Werner M. Herrmann

Acknowledgements

We wish to express our gratitude to *Frauke Alashe, Maria-Sophie Glücklich, Marion Hofmann, Margot Hübenthal, Helga Lehmann, Heide Niehues, Monika Rosanowski, Gisela Waldeck* and *Gabriele Zablonski* for their most valuable assistance during the implementation of this book.

We would also like to thank Mr. *Rudolf Lohaus* for his excellent work done in the evaluation of difficult biometric data. Special thanks are dedicated to *Horst Buchmann,* Cappenberg, Dr. *Thomas Karger, Rolf Steinebrunner* and *Anke Rogal,* Basle, for their honest encouragement and support.

The Board of Editors

Adv. Pharmacother., vol. 1, pp. 1–3 (Karger, Basel 1982)

Introduction

W.-D. Bussmann

Center of Internal Medicine, Department of Cardiology, University Clinic of the Johann Wolfgang Goethe University, Frankfurt am Main, FRG

The first scientific workshop in Kronberg, 2 years ago, was dedicated to the dosage of nitrates. As a result, we are now using higher daily doses of isosorbide dinitrate ranging from 120 to 480 mg or more per day. Dr. *Schneider* from our group recently demonstrated, that a dose-response relationship exists for antianginal activity of isosorbide dinitrate. The patients received 5–80 mg ISDN 6 times daily, each dose for 1 week. ST-segment depression during exercise decreased gradually when the dose was increased. 80 mg ISDN resulted in 70% decrease of ST-segment depression.

Plasma levels of the parent substance isosorbide dinitrate and the two mononitrates were analyzed. Despite the known first-pass effect the parent substance as well as the metabolites increased when the dose was augmented from 5 to 80 mg. The good dose-response relationship suggests that the antianginal properties of isosorbide dinitrate during chronic therapy is not blunted after 1 week. Tolerance seems to be unlikely [*Schneider* et al., 1981].

Last year during the 2nd workshop, we discussed the usefulness of isosorbide-5′-mononitrate as a new preparation and came to the conclusion that 5′-mononitrate has little advantage over the parent substance [*Kaltenbach* et al., 1980].

This third workshop is in a certain sense a step backward: From the mononitrates to the oldest of the trinitrates: nitroglycerin. Sublingual nitroglycerin and, for 8 years, intravenous nitroglycerin have been used widely, but oral or buccal nitroglycerin are viewed with scepticism. The drug list drawn up by the Transparenz-Kommission of the Bundesgesundheitsamt, the German Federal Health Office, maintains that slow-release nitroglycerin tablets are probably ineffective because of the first-pass effect and the low dose used. Nitroglycerin in tablet form is not or only rarely used in Germany and in other European countries. The substance is, however, used in the United States to a certain extent, and with success. Our patients are treated with large doses of isosorbide dinitrate, which has been investigated extensively in recent years.

In the use of buccal or oral nitroglycerin, an effective way of releasing the drug slowly is of considerable importance. Slow release nitroglycerin tablets are marketed in Germany in the form of pellets, which dissolve during the passage through the intestines. A new form is to be discussed here. Nitroglycerin is incorporated in a modified cellulose structure, which releases the drug when it comes into contact with water. The release of nitroglycerin from the buccal form seems to be comparable to an intravenous infusion of the drug.

The workshop hopes to answer some of the following questions: (1) Is buccal and is oral nitroglycerin an effective way to treat patients with angina pectoris? We have to clearly distinguish between the two, since buccal absorption is rapid and presents no problems. Oral administration, however, is subject to a marked first-pass effect by the liver and also problems due to absorption in the intestines. (2) Are the results comparable to the favorable results, which have been achieved with dinitrates? (3) What is the dose range of these drugs? Do we need the same large doses for the oral route as we do with isosorbide dinitrate? (4) The duration of action should be discussed in detail. (5) One of the most important questions today however should be: The buccal controlled release tablet. What is the advantage of such a preparation, what are the pharmacokinetic-hemodynamic effects?

With a buccal tablet a patient is able to stop his own 'infusion' of nitroglycerin in a way comparable to the newer forms of transdermal nitroglycerin. Is it an important feature to position the tablet in the mouth and to stop and restart nitroglycerin release? What about the patient's compliance about having a buccal tablet left in his mouth for 2–3 h? The presentations and the discussion during the workshop elucidate a new type of a nitroglycerin preparation, allowing us to infuse nitroglycerin over a number of hours easily by a buccal tablet, left in the patients buccal pouch.

References

1 Schneider, W.; Stahl, B.; Bussmann, W.-D.; Kaltenbach, M.: Dose-relationship in the treatment of angina pectoris with oral isosorbide dinitrate (Abstract). Eur. Heart J. *2:* suppl. A, p. 94 (1981).

2 Kaltenbach, M.; Bussmann, W.-D.; Schrey, R. (ed.): Mononitrat. Workshop, Kronberg 1980, pp. 1–143 (Wolf & Sohn, Munich 1981).

W.-D. Bussmann, MD, Professor of Medicine, Center of Internal Medicine, Department of Cardiology, University Clinic of the Johann Wolfgang Goethe University, D-6000 Frankfurt a.M. (FRG)

Adv. Pharmacother., vol. 1, pp. 4–16 (Karger, Basel 1982)

Nitroglycerin and Long-Acting Nitrates: A Contemporary Perspective

Jonathan Abrams

Division of Cardiology, University of New Mexico School of Medicine, Albuquerque, N. Mex., USA

More than 100 years ago *William Murrell* used an oral nitroglycerin solution in a patient with angina pectoris. Since that report sublingual nitroglycerin (GTN) has become the mainstay of the acute treatment of chest pain caused by myocardial ischemia, and nitrates in various formulations have been given to hundreds of thousands of patients around the world. At the present time rational nitrate therapy is enjoying a renaissance, with a widening clinical role for these agents and an increasing flexibility and efficacy of nitrate delivery systems. This paper will document the somewhat circuitous history of nitrate use and will emphasize current clinical and research indications for these agents. In addition the presently available nitrate formulations and dosage recommendations will be reviewed.

Historical Evolution of Nitrate Therapy

Denigration of Long-Acting Nitrates. Although numerous oral nitrate esters have been available to clinicians for many years, by the late 1960s and early 1970s long-acting nitrate preparations were universally condemned and little utilized. Why was this disillusion so widespread? (1) Careful clinical investigations were unable to demonstrate a clear-cut efficacy for nitrate esters compared to sublingual nitroglycerin in the treatment of angina. Many early studies showed positive results, but a review of 59 investigations carried out between 1952 and 1972 concluded that the majority of positive studies were poorly designed with inadequate controls, rare use of placebo, and lack of an appropriate double-blind crossover protocol [1]. When only those trials that met appropriate criteria were analyzed, there was at best equivocal evidence for nitrate efficacy in the treatment of angina. (2) A series of elegant animal experiments carried out by *Needleman* and co-workers at Washington University in St. Louis clearly indicated that the metabolism of orally administered nitrates is so rapid and complete as to preclude the appearance of effective concentrations in the systemic circulation [2, 3]. Using a rat model *Needleman* [3] demonstrated that organic nitrate esters are quickly degraded by hepatic organic nitrate glutathione reductase activity, literally within minutes. Virtually none of the parent nitrate appeared in the blood following the potent first pass metabolism. In addition, it was found that the most potent nitrates with respect to vasodilator activity were the most rapidly metabolized, suggesting that those compounds that were most likely to work were precisely the ones that would have the most difficulty 'escaping' hepatic clearance [2]. When the same nitrates were introduced into the systemic circulation bypassing the liver, vasodilation occurred, but if an equivalent dose was given directly into the portal vein, no biologic activity was noted. As recently as 1976 *Needleman* [4] asked, 'Why, then, do clinicians and other workers advocate the use of oral nitrates as long-acting prophylactic medication?' *Needleman's* work was widely publicized and had an enormous impact on clinical investigators. Many other prominent scientists and pharmacologists were extremely vocal in their condemnation of long-acting nitrates. (3) The dosages of nitrate esters used in early clinical studies were small, particularly compared to modern-day usage. It is likely that orally administered nitrates were given in insufficient quantity to reach the systemic circulation after hepatic degradation. Even if a biologic effect was noted, it persisted for such a short time that it seemed little better than sublingual GTN. It is likely that the advent of beta blocker therapy for angina and the dramatic proliferation of coronary bypass surgery in the early 1970s distracted clinicians from any lingering interest in nitrates as an important modality for the control of angina. Long-acting nitrates were clearly out of favor.

Resurgence of Long-Acting Nitrates. In the past 4–5 years, there has been a remarkable turnabout in the attitude towards the use of nitrates in clinical practice. This symposium, as well as others held in the last 2 years, attest to the widespread interest in nitrates that exists not only in Germany but throughout the world. Why is this so? Again, a brief look at history is in order. A number of studies in the mid-1970s were carried out that met appropriate criteria for properly conducted angina protocols and more importantly, higher doses of nitrates were employed than had been used in the past. The results were uniformally positive [5]. In 1974, *Reichek* et al. [6] reported an investigation utilizing GTN ointment in patients with angina.

This serial treadmill study documented prolonged efficacy of topically applied GTN and some believe this was the first clear evidence that long-acting nitrate preparations do work. However, topical nitroglycerin administration does not involve hepatic metabolism. Subsequently, successful investigations have been reported using large doses of oral isosorbide dinitrate (ISDN) or GTN demonstrating prolonged anginal protection, improvement in myocardial ischemia as assessed by S-T response, and increased exercise performance [5, 7]. It thus became evident that our concepts of long-acting nitrate therapy again had to be revised.

Major new evidence of support for the efficacy of oral nitrate therapy appeared following the introduction vasodilator therapy for congestive heart failure. In the mid-1970s many investigators around the world looked for drugs that would reduce left ventricular (LV) afterload and preload, resulting in improved myocardial performance as well as a fall in LV filling pressure in patients with deranged LV function. Nitrates were studied in numerous centers and were found to be extremely effective in reducing pulmonary artery and capillary wedge pressures, often with a modest improvement in stroke volume and cardiac output. Patients in heart failure tolerate nitrate preparations extremely well. Nitrates quickly became the agents of choice for the treatment of 'backwards' failure, with improvement in the signs and symptoms of pulmonary congestion. Oral administration of GTN, ISDN, and pentaerythrital tetranitrate (PETN) have all been shown to lower LV filling pressure in these patients for many hours [8]. Reflex tachycardia and hypotension is rarely seen. It has become evident that rather large doses of nitrates are required in congestive heart failure, probably greater than those needed in most cases of angina pectoris. In addition, there is suggestive evidence that these higher doses are required in order to provide afterload reduction and a fall in systemic vascular resistance, whereas LV preload (venous capacitance) is reduced at lower dosage.

Many investigations have demonstrated prolonged physiologic activity of long-acting nitrates, documenting sustained bioavailability and pharmacologic action for periods of up to 2–8 h [5, 8]. In addition, recent utilization of plasma nitrate levels has firmly documented that sustained therapeutic concentrations of GTN and ISDN persist for many hours after oral and topical administration [9, 10]. This work certainly lays to rest any lingering doubts regarding hepatic degradation precluding adequate amounts of nitrate from reaching the systemic circulation after oral ingestion of nitrate esters. Presumably, a large oral dose literally overwhelms the liver's capacity to completely metabolize the nitrate.

Nitrate Blood Levels. The advent of an accurate and sensitive gas chromatographic technique for measurement of nitroglycerin and nitrate esters represents a major advance in our understanding of nitrate pharmacology and bioeffectiveness. Assays of GTN and ISDN have shown a good correlation between acute dosing and plasma levels and physiologic effects [9, 10]. Plasma levels increase with increasing dosage, and the time course of nitrate activity corresponds with the blood levels of the parent compound of GTN and ISDN. However, serious questions have been raised by some nitrate blood level data. In chronic repetitive dosing with ISDN there is a less clear and often absent relationship between the plasma concentration and physiologic actions [11]. In addition, it seems clear that patients have varying sensitivity to nitrate compounds; some subjects are extremely sensitive and others are relatively or completely resistant to the effects of nitrate. We know little about this phenomenon. Preliminary data with ISDN suggest a differing rate of plasma clearance in patients who are more or less responsive to the drug [12]. In heart failure, a subset of patients has been identified who do not respond to GTN whether given intravenously or topically [13]. These individuals appear to be the most severely affected, often with peripheral edema and hepatic congestion. This suggests target organ resistance, which may or may not be susceptible to therapeutic interventions. One study demonstrated a definite response to GTN only after diuretic treatment [14].

Nitrate Tolerance. Studies of nitrate tolerance using blood levels indicate that increased degradation or clearance of nitrates is not a factor. This vexing problem is still clouded by conflicting data as to whether or not nitrate tolerance is a clinical reality. Work from Ontario, Canada, strongly suggests that tolerance to ISDN is rapidly induced after only a few doses, resulting in a decreased duration of effectiveness of the parent compound and the loss of some but not all of the biological effects of the ISDN [11]. Many other studies have been unable to document clinically important nitrate tolerance [15]. Clearly, more work on the question of tolerance is needed.

Current Indications for Nitroglycerin and Long-Acting Nitrates (table I)

The use of nitrate esters has been considerably expanded in recent years. These drugs are still the first line of defense in patients with chronic, effort-induced or secondary angina. GTN acts by decreasing myocardial oxygen demands [16] and possibly in part by increasing blood flow to ischemic zones

Table I. Clinical and investigational indications for nitroglycerin and long-acting nitrates

Cardiac
Exertional angina pectoris
Accelerating angina pectoris
Chronic congestive heart failure
Acute heart failure or pulmonary edema
Adjunct therapy of mitral and aortic regurgitation
Treatment and prevention of coronary vasospasm
Variant (Prinzmetal's) angina
Unstable angina pectoris
Fibrinolytic therapy for acute myocardial infarction
Percutaneous transluminal angioplasty
Acute myocardial infarction
Reduction of infarct size
Reduction in early and late phase ventricular dysrhythmia
Pain control
Lowering of blood pressure in hypertensive subjects
Intervention left ventriculography
Non-cardiac
Treatment of diffuse esophageal spasm
Reduction of intraocular pressure in open angle glaucoma
Control of blood pressure during neurosurgical procedures and general anesthesia

of the myocardium [17]. In patients with classic angina, exercise performance is enhanced and LV function may be improved with effective doses of nitrates that reduce myocardial ischemia.

Congestive Heart Failure. Nitrates are effective adjunctive agents in the treatment of acute and chronic congestive heart failure. They work both through preload and afterload reduction, with substantial falls in LV filling pressure and pulmonary artery pressure and often an increase in cardiac index. Patients most likely to benefit from nitrates are those with a high systemic vascular resistance, low cardiac output, and high LV filling pressure [8]. Nitrates are often used in conjunction with a vasodilator that has major action on the arterial system, such as hydralazine, whose 'afterload unloading' action is far more potent than GTN and results in a large increase in cardiac output.

Acute Myocardial Infarction. Nitroglycerin in various formulations is very beneficial in acute myocardial infarction. When given in the early hours after the onset of infarction, it appears that eventual myocardial infarction size may be reduced [18]. Pulmonary capillary wedge pressure declines, usually with no major change or a slight increase in cardiac output and a fall in systemic vascular resistance. As expected, patients with a high LV filling pressure benefit most. Human [18] and animal [19] experiments have shown a decrease in acute ischemia and predicted infarct size, although these results have not been reproduced by all investigators [20]. Several studies have documented an elevation in the ventricular fibrillation threshold [21] and a reduction in acute [22] and late phase ventricular arrhythmias [23] following myocardial infarction. A recent investigation demonstrated that sublingual GTN in repetitive large doses was somewhat more effective than intravenous morphine in relieving infarction pain and also appeared to prevent the evolution to Q-wave infarction in some patients [24].

While nitrates appear to have an important role in the treatment of acute myocardial infarction, this mode of therapy is still investigational. Almost all studies have been carried out with intravenous GTN; the precise dosage required is unclear and invasive monitoring is mandatory. GTN may be harmful to some patients with acute ischemia if there is decreased myocardial perfusion resulting from systemic hypotension. Reflex tachycardia could be deleterious, and the combination of a fall in central aortic pressure and increased heart rate could result in infarct extension. These potential life-threatening side effects may ultimately limit the widespread application of nitrates in acute myocardial infarction.

Nitrates and Coronary Vasospasm. Another major area for nitrate utilization is the treatment of coronary artery spasm, a subject which has been a focus of cardiologists around the world in the past several years. The work of *Maseri* et al. [25] from Italy has crystallized our view of the importance of coronary vasomotor tone in a number of coronary syndromes. It is now believed that coronary vasospasm may play a role in some cases of effort-induced angina [26], as well as 'routine' acute myocardial infarction [25, 27]. Many investigators believe that accelerating or unstable angina and some atypical pain syndromes are related to coronary vasospasm [25]. Although nitrate therapy had been the mainstay of treatment for vasospasm in the past, present evidence indicates that calcium antagonists such as nifedipine and diltiazem may ultimately replace nitrates as the treatment of choice for coronary vasospasm. It is still unclear whether these new agents are in fact more effective than nitroglycerin preparations in equivalent dosage.

There are several other clinical situations where nitrates have been used and appear to be efficacious (table I). Most of these studies are preliminary but indicate the wide spectrum of disorders where nitroglycerin and its congeners can be extremely beneficial.

High-Dose Nitrate Therapy

Recent investigations have clearly shown that far larger doses of GTN and long-acting nitrates are needed than had previously been utilized. There is suggestive evidence that heart failure patients require greater amounts of nitrate than subjects with well-preserved LV function. Afterload reduction may be seen only at higher doses in patients with major derangement of LV function [28].

One should not conclude that GTN or ISDN is ineffective until at least 13–19.5 mg of oral NTG have been given or 20–40 mg of oral ISDN have been administrated without beneficial effect. Even higher dosages have been used [29]. Table II lists recommended doses for standard nitrate preparations. Nitrate therapy must be initiated with low doses and increased judiciously. Limiting side effects can usually be treated by temporarily cutting back the dosage. Acceptable tolerance to headaches generally will develop in the first 1–2 weeks.

Nitrate Delivery Systems

There is no evidence that one nitrate ester has a significantly different clinical or physiologic effect than any other [30]. Some clinicians feel that ISDN is more likely to produce debilitating headaches than oral GTN. Many efforts are currently under way to improve nitrate formulations in order to provide sustained bioavailable drug levels. I will not deal with the new buccal tablet, which is discussed at length in this symposium. Table III lists delivery systems currently available for GTN and ISDN. Many of these preparations are not yet available in all countries. In addition to GTN ointment, GTN-impregnated disks for topical administration are being tested that will deliver a fixed amount of GTN over protracted time without the mess and uncertainty of nitrate dose of the ointment. Topical ISDN is effective but not available in the United States. A GTN nasal spray has been tested in patients with angina. Oral sustained-action formulations of GTN and ISDN have been used for some years.

Table II. Dosage recommendations for long-acting nitrates. Individual sensitivity to nitrate effects and duration of action is extremely variable from subject to subject. Patients with congestive heart failure in general require larger dosage of nitrates

Drug	Dosage	Duration of action, h
Oral nitroglycerin	6.5–19.5 mg every 4–6 h	4–6
2% nitroglycerin ointment	0.5–2 in. (1.3–5 cm; 7.5–30 mg) every 4–6 h	3–6
Isosorbide dinitrate		
Sublingual	2.5–10 mg every 2–4 h	1.5–3
Oral	10–60 mg every 4–6 h	4–8
Chewable	5–10 mg every 2–4 h	2–3
Oral pentaerythritol tetranitrate	40–80 mg every 4–6 h	3–5

Table III. Nitrate delivery systems. Note that some of these formulations are not commercially available. Some are available in certain countries and not in others

Sublingual	GTN	ISDN
Oral	GTN	ISDN
Chewable		ISDN
Topical ointment	GTN	ISDN
Topical Disc	GTN	
Nasal spray	GTN	
Oral spray	GTN	
Buccal tablet	GTN	
Intravenous	GTN	ISDN

GTN = nitroglycerin; ISDN = isosorbide dinitrate.

Conclusions

GTN and long-acting nitrates have a definite role in the therapy of effort-angina, vasospastic angina, and severe congestive heart failure. Nitrates have been used extensively in studies of acute myocardial infarction and appear to have a range of beneficial actions in this important clinical entity. Although still investigational, it is likely that GTN will become routine in the treatment of selective patients with acute myocardial infarction in the years ahead.

High dosages of nitrates are frequently required, especially in heart failure and 'refractory' angina. Present dosage recommendations far exceed amounts used in the past. There is increasing data utilizing nitrate blood levels, which have demonstrated that nitrate esters are bioavailable for many hours after oral or topical administration. Much more needs to be learned about the relationships of nitrate levels to physiologic actions, patient sensitivity, and the problem of nitrate tolerance. Finally, clinicians will have available an increasingly sophisticated and effective array of nitrate delivery systems that will allow more rational nitrate therapy in the years ahead.

References

1 Stipe, A.A.; Fink, G.B.: Prophylactic therapy of angina pectoris with organic nitrates, relationship of drug efficacy and clinical experimental design. J. clin. Pharm. *13:* 244–250 (1973).

2 Needleman, P.; Lang, E.; Johnson, E.M.: Organic nitrates: relationship between biotransformation and rational angina pectoris therapy. J. Pharm. exp. Ther. *181:* 489 (1972).

3 Needleman, P.: Biotransformation of organic nitrates; in Needleman, Handbook of experimental pharmacology, vol. 40, pp. 57–95 (Springer, Berlin 1975).

4 Needleman, P.: Efficacy of long-acting nitrates. Am. J. Cardiol. *38:* 400–402 (1976).

5 Abrams, J.: Usefulness of long-acting nitrates in cardiovascular disease. Am. J. Med. *64:* 183–185 (1978).

6 Reichek, N.; Goldstein, R.E.; Redwood, D.R.; Epstein, S.E.: Sustained effects of nitroglycerin ointment in patients with angina pectoris. Circulation *50:* 348 (1974).

7 Danahy, D.T.; Aronow, W.S.: Hemodynamics and antianginal effects of high-dose oral isosorbide dinitrate after chronic use. Circulation *56:* 205–212 (1977).

8 Abrams, J.: Pharmacology of nitroglycerin and long-acting nitrates and their usefulness in the treatment of chronic congestive heart failure; in Gould, Reddy, Vasodilator therapy for cardiac disorders, pp. 129–167 (Futura, Mount Kisco 1979).

9 Girre, C.; Crouzette, J.; Fournier, P.E.: Taux plasmatiques de nitroglycerin après administration orale et percutanée. Nouv. Presse méd. *9:* 2433–2436 (1980).

10 Thadani, U.; Fung, H.L.; Darke, A.C.; Parker, J.O.: Oral isosorbide dinitrate in the treatment of angina pectoris. Circulation *62:* 491–497 (1980).

11 Thadani, U.; Manyari, D.; Parker, J.O.; Fung, H.L.: Tolerance to the circulatory effects of oral isosorbide nitrate. Circulation *61:* 526–535 (1980).

12 Fung, H.L.; McNiff, E.F.; Ruggirello, D.; Darke, A.; Thadani, U.; Parker, J.O.: Pharmokinetics and relationships to pharmacologic effects of isosorbide dinitrate after acute and chronic dosing (Abstract). 3rd Int. Symp. of Nitrates, Monte Carlo 1980, p. 76.

13 Armstrong, P.W.; Armstrong, J.A.; Marks, G.S.: Pharmokinetic-hemodynamic studies of intravenous nitroglycerin in congestive heart failure. Circulation *62:* 160–166 (1980).

14 Magrini, F.; Niarchos, A.P.: Ineffectiveness of sublingual nitroglycerin in acute ventricular failure in the presence of massive peripheral edema. Am. J. Cardiol. *45:* 841–847 (1980).

15 Abrams, J.: Nitrate tolerance and dependence. Am. Heart J. *99:* 113–123 (1980).

16 Vatner, S.F.; Heyndricks, G.R.: Mechanism of action of nitroglycerin: coronary, cardiac and systemic effects; in Needleman, Handbook of experimental pharmacology, vol. 40, pp. 131–161 (Springer, Berlin 1975).

17 Horwitz, L.D.; Gorlin, R.; Taylor, W.J.; Kemp, H.G.: Effects of nitroglycerin on regional myocardial blood flow in coronary artery disease. J. clin. Invest. *50:* 1578–1584 (1971).

18 Bussmann, W.-D.; Passek, D.; Seidel, W.; Kaltenbach, M.: Reduction of CK and CK-MB indexes of infarct size by intravenous nitroglycerin. Circulation *63:* 615–622 (1981).

19 Judgutt, B.; Hutchins, G.; Bulkley, B.H.; Becker, L.: Reduction of infarct size by intravenous nitroglycerin infusion in conscious dogs (Abstract). Circulation *58:* suppl. 2, pp. II–98 (1978).

20 Fukuyama, T.; Roberts, R.: Lack of effect of nitroglycerin on morphometrically and enzymatically estimated infarct size (Abstract). Circulation *58:* suppl. 2, pp. II–98 (1978).

21 Kent, K.M.; Smith, E.R.; Redwood, D.R.; Epstein, S.E.: Beneficial electrophysiologic effects of nitroglycerin during acute myocardial infarction. Am. J. Cardiol. *35:* 513–520 (1974).

22 Mihalick, M.J.; Rasmussen, S.; Knoebel, S.B.: The effect of nitroglycerin on premature ventricular complexes in acute myocardial infarction (Abstract). Am. J. Cardiol. *33:* 157 (1974).

23 Becker, L.; Bulkley, B.H.; Flaherty, J.; Weiss, J.; Pitt, B.; Gerstenblith, G.; Llewelyn, M.; Weisfeldt, M.: Reduction of late complex ventricular arrythmias by nitroglycerin in patients with acute myocardial infarction: results of a prospective randomized trial (Abstract). Circulation *58:* suppl. 2, pp. II–61 (1978).

24 Kim, Y.I.; Williams, J.F.: Relief of chest pain and reduction of Q-wave evolution in acute myocardial infarction by large dose sublingual nitroglycerin (Abstract). Am. J. Cardiol. *45:* 483 (1980).

25 Maseri, A.; L'Abbate, A.; Chierchia, S.; Parodi, O.; Severi, S.; Biagini, A.; Distante, A.; Marzilli, M.; Ballestra, A.M.: Significance of spasm and the pathogenesis of ischemic heart disease. Am. J. Cardiol. *44:* 788–792 (1979).

26 Yasue, H.; Omote, S.; Takizawa, A.; Nagao, M.; Miwa, K.; Tanaka, S.: Exertional angina pectoris caused by coronary arterial spasm: effects of various drugs. Am. J. Cardiol. *43:* 647–652 (1979).

27 Oliva, P.B.; Breckenridge, J.C.: Arteriographic evidence of coronary arterial spasm in acute myocardial infarction. Circulation *56:* 366–374 (1977).

28 Baligadoo, S.; Chiche, P.: Les dérivés nitrés sont ils efficaces par la voie orale? Nouv. Presse méd. *9:* 2419–2428 (1980).

29 Shane, S.J.: High dose oral isosorbide dinitrate and ischemic heart pain. Can. Fam. Phys. *19:* 61 (1973).

30 Abrams, J.: Nitroglycerin and long-acting nitrates. New Engl. J. Med. *302:* 1234–1237 (1980).

J. Abrams, MD, Professor of Medicine, Chief, Division of Cardiology,
University of New Mexico School of Medicine, Albuquerque, NM 87131 (USA)

Discussion

Chairman: *H.-L. Fung*

Gleichmann: Dr. *Abrams,* I wonder if you could comment on the at least in Germany controversial question of tolerance? If there is a loss of therapeutic efficacy during long-term treatment with isosorbide dinitrate?

Abrams: It's a subject of great importance, one which I have looked at rather carefully, although not through any personal investigations. The work that Dr. *Fung* has participated in indirectly from Dr. *Parker's* laboratory in Ontario is of course I think what you are referring to. All I can say is that their experimental design is very elaborate, and they have looked at this question I think more carefully than any other investigators and have found that very rapidly the administration of isosorbide to patients with angina results in an attenuation or a blunting of the heart rate and blood pressure responses and a reduction of the angina protection time from something like 6 down to 2 h. Other workers, as I'm sure you are aware, who have looked at this question recently have not been able to demonstrate such tolerance or tachyphylaxis. I think the question is up for grabs. There are many other studies that have been conducted over the last several years that do not seem to show any loss of potency. I have talked to almost every nitrate investigator – at least in the United States – about this, and they claim they do not see it. Nevertheless, the work from Canada looks at it more carefully and systematically. I think it is entirely possible that their design has picked something that has simply been missed by others. I don't know the ultimate answer to this. I think we have to keep our eyes open for this. I wonder if in Germany there has been some or any work that sheds light on this?

Bussmann: I would like to comment on this paper from Canada. I don't think that what Dr. *Thadani* and Dr. *Parker* elaborated means tolerance. They only looked at hemodynamic parameters. Heart rate and blood pressure in the standing position. If you swallow 120 mg of isosorbide dinitrate, then the blood pressure goes down in the standing position. This has nothing to do with the anti-anginal effect. We didn't find any tolerance, as you saw from my slide. There was a dose-dependent decrease in exercise-induced ischemia after 1 week. We continued therapy for 4 weeks with the high dose, and we found no attenuation of anginal activity. Blunting of the hemodynamic effect is normal since counterregulation takes place, even though a decrease in blood pressure to 80 mm Hg every day is impossible. In these circumstances counterregulation plays an important role. But this has nothing to do with tolerance to the anti-anginal effect.

Abrams: There is work, as I think some of you may be aware, animal work going back to the 1930s and 1940s showing that blood pressure responses are blunted very rapidly after nitrates. In fact, one can make a strip of aorta and make it totally unresponsive to nitroglycerin by pretreatment with nitrates. So I think the blood pressure and heart rate information is certainly not new nor is it surprising. The duration of angina protection from isosorbide was reduced in Dr. *Parker's* paper in a serial protocol using multiple treadmill tests from 6 down to 2 h but there still was protection and increased time on the treadmill and decreased ischemia at 120 min. So it is not just the blood pressure.

Fung: Let me speak on behalf of my collaborators, Dr. *Parker* and Dr. *Thadani.* Yes I think we have found circulatory tolerance. I think that point perhaps is not as controversial as the claim of anti-anginal tolerance. The paper that Dr. *Abrams* referred to I believe will be appearing in the *American Journal of Cardiology* which shows that the treadmill walking was reduced from 6 h during acute dosing to about 2 h during chronic dosing. My involvement with those papers was through the pharmacokinetic analysis, and I cannot speak to the detail or the validity of the clinical testing, but from my impression, I think the tolerance question as Dr. *Abrams* has

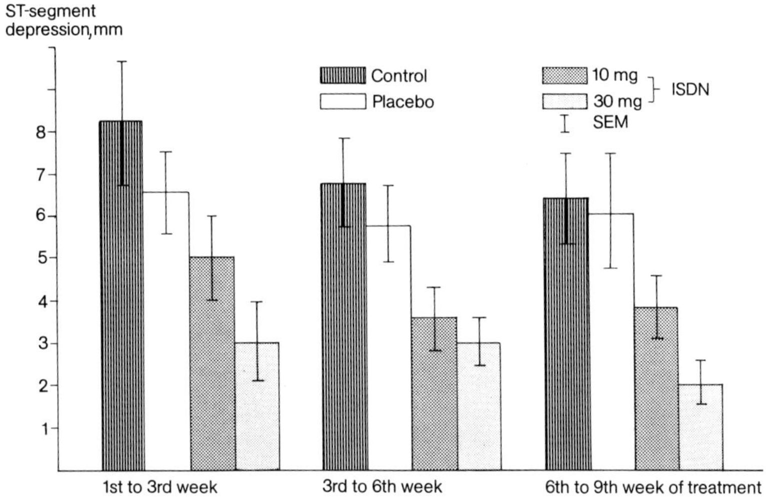

Fig. 1. Long-term effect of ISDN (n= 10).

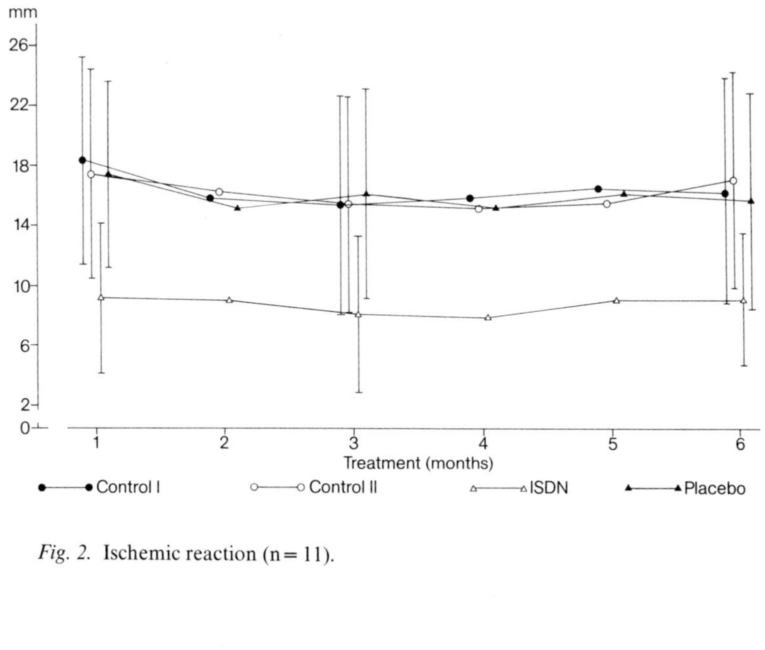

Fig. 2. Ischemic reaction (n= 11).

pointed out is a very complex one. It involves practically different methodology and different patient populations. I think it may be difficult to state whether there is tolerance or there is no tolerance. Perhaps it is more proper to state that there is tolerance in what parameters in what patients, under what conditions or dosing I think these qualifications perhaps are necessary to address the question of tolerance as such, rather than just whether or not there is tolerance.

Reichek: I would like to make some comments on the issue of tolerance. The first is to underscore Dr. *Bussmann's* point which I think is essential and which comes up time and again in trying to evaluate the literature on any aspect of the nitrates. The end point selected for examining physiologic response is very much a determinant of one's impression of the duration of the effect of any dose of any particular agent. It's essential to remind ourselves repeatedly that if what we're interested in practically, is angina prophylaxis that none of these other end points can be substituted for it in a satisfactory way. The second point I wanted to make was that the problems inherent in protocol design for determining whether there is attenuation of anti-anginal efficacy, during chronic administration were very formidable. I'm not certain that it is going to be possible to solve all of them. For example, one can look at the acute dose response during chronic therapy and that is necessary, but not sufficient to establish efficacy because one does not know what the effect of the background milieu of repeated administration of doses over the days prior to study is on the manifest effect of the single dose. It's very hard to design a study that addresses all of the factors that goes into this question of tolerance. Moreover, if one examines the industrial toxicology literature on nitrates, which is really rather extensive and has a very long history going back to the 1890s I guess, it is very apparent that the tolerance to virtually any pharmacologic effect of nitrates can be produced in man with sufficient intensity of exposure. I think, therefore, the question for the future will become: Will we be required to use such large amounts of nitrate agents to obtain the desired therapeutic effects that we will begin to enter the range where we produce the kinds of tolerance that the industrial toxicologists have documented repeatedly.

Becker: In reference to the topic of tolerance we did a study in 1976 in patients with evidence of coronary arteriosclerosis, who were on a daily dosis of 100 mg ISDN. In a double-blind randomized cross-over study, we performed repeated exercise tests before and after 10, 30 mg ISDN or placebo over a period of 9 weeks. We saw that there were no signs of tolerance in this group of patients investigated. Under a daily dose of 100 mg ISDN an additional dose of 10 or 30 mg ISDN led to an improvement of ST-segment depression, which was not attenuated after a 9-week treatment.

We just ended another study in patients who were under 160 mg ISDN daily. We did in the same manner repeated exercise tests over a period of 6 months. We found no signs of tolerance during this time (fig. 1, 2).

Adv. Pharmacother., vol. 1, pp. 17–25 (Karger, Basel 1982)

Design and Evaluation of Sustained Release Formulations for Oral and Buccal Administration

S.S. Davis[a], *P.B. Daly*[a], *J.W. Kennerley*[a], *M. Frier*[b], *J.G. Hardy*[b], *C.G. Wilson*[c]

[a] Department of Pharmacy, University of Nottingham; [b] Department of Medical Physics, Queen's Medical Centre; [c] Department of Physiology and Pharmacology, The Medical School, University of Nottingham, Nottingham, England

Introduction

Sustained release dosage forms can offer advantages over conventional preparations; for example improved patient compliance, reduced side-effects and extended action [1]. Claims for an improvement in therapy are usually based upon the advantage of continuous therapeutic blood levels as opposed to an intermittent or 'peak and valley' pattern [2]. Glyceryl trinitrate has a very short biological half-life (0.55 h) and therefore an extended duration of action is of considerable therapeutic benefit. Glyceryl trinitrate can be administered in various ways including the oral, sublingual or buccal routes. The last two have been popular because the drug is rapidly absorbed.

Many techniques are available for the design of sustained release products. These have been reviewed by *Notari* [2] and *Ballard* [3]. The two most popular approaches are the use of pellet systems (as capsules and tablets) and matrix systems (as tablets); both have been used for glyceryl trinitrate [1, 4, 5].

Pellet systems are multiparticulate dosage forms where the drug is incorporated into pellets, beads or microcapsules. The pellets are coated with suitable polymers, sometimes of different thicknesses, and these control the rate of release of the drug. The mechanism of release can be via degradation of the polymer in the body fluids or the permeation of the drug through the polymer layer. Pellet systems are complicated to manufacture but have the advantage that the dosage is distributed well in the gastrointestinal tract and consequently drug release is not dependent on gastric residence [6].

Matrix systems take the appearance of conventional tablets but the drug is entrapped in a slowly eroding non-disintegrating tablet base, such as wax, polymer or gum. The liberation of the drug depends inter alia on the type and amount of matrix material. For gum systems release is dependent on the diffusion of the drug through a layer of hydrated gum rather than dissolution of the gum or penetration of water provided the hydrated gelatinous layer remains intact. Matrix systems are normally much easier to prepare than pellet systems. They have the disadvantage that the release rate can depend sometimes upon the transit of the product down the gastro-intestinal tract. Sustained release products for buccal administration need to be in the form of a non-disintegrating matrix unit. *Kutscher and Zigarelli* [7] have discussed the merits of incorporating drugs into slowly dissolving lozenges held in the buccal cavity and *Ritschel and Clother* [5] have described a two-layered buccal tablet of glyceryl trinitrate.

A problem that is unique to sustained release dosage forms is demonstrating a sustained effect [2], and this is more difficult than might be anticipated. Studies can be conducted in vitro and the release of the drug into dissolution media of different characteristic (e.g. pH) can be followed. However, the release of the drug in the body may not correlate well with the in vitro situation. A number of reports on the deleterious effect of physiological variables and food on the release of drugs from sustained release dosage forms have appeared recently [8, 9]. An obvious way to evaluate a sustained release product is to measure the appearance of the drug in the systemic circulation or monitor a physiological variable to determine a pharmacological or clinical response. Such techniques do not give an insight into the disintegration and dissolution behaviour of the dosage form within the gastro-intestinal tract. Other appropriate methods have included radiographic studies on tablets containing radio-opaque materials. This technique has limitations and recently we have employed gamma scintigraphy to monitor externally the position of sustained release dosages in the body and the release of marker substances therefrom [10, 11]. The sustained release system described in the present communication is a matrix tablet made from a modified hydroxypropylmethylcellulose (Synchron) [12]. Practical considerations prevent labelling of the drug directly with a gamma-emitting radionuclide, and the non-absorbable water-soluble chelate ^{99m}Tc-labelled diethylenetriamine-pentaacetic acid (^{99m}Tc-DTPA) has been used to model the behaviour of the drug. Studies conducted in vitro have demonstrated that ^{99m}Tc-DTPA has similar release characteristics to water-soluble compounds.

Materials and Methods

Hydroxypropyl methylcellulose (Synchron) was obtained from Pharmax Limited, α-lactose monohydrate from Whey Products, *D*-mannitol from Cambrian Chemicals, and DTPA from CIS Biomedical Products.

Preparation of Tablets

^{99m}Tc pertechnetate in 2 ml saline was obtained by elution from a generator (Amersham International) and was used to prepare ^{99m}Tc-DTPA [11]. Three different types of tablet were prepared.

1. Oral sustained release tablets: ^{99m}Tc-DTPA 30 mg, Synchron 270 mg (total activity 4.4 MBq); compaction pressure 165 MNm^{-2}, 10-mm diameter flat punches.

2. Sublingual (rapidly dissolving): ^{99m}Tc-DTPA 2.5 mg, α-Lactose monohydrate 72.5 mg, *D*-Mannitol 75 mg (total activity 0.4 MBq); compaction pressure 195 MNm^{-2}, 7-mm diameter biconcave punches.

3. Buccal sustained release: ^{99m}Tc-DTPA 2.5 mg, α-Lactose monohydrate 72.5 mg, Synchron 75 mg (activity and compaction as for formulation 2).

All tablets were compressed on an instrumented Manesty F3 machine.

In vitro Evaluation

The in vitro release of ^{99m}Tc-DTPA from the oral tablets was measured using the USP rotating basket method at 100 revolutions per minute using media at pH 1.0. Samples of the dissolution medium were removed periodically and assayed with a gamma counter.

In vivo Evaluation

The oral sustained release tablets were given to 4 healthy male volunteers. The subjects had fasted overnight and during the study they were allowed a light lunch. During the course of the study each subject swallowed two doses of 2 MBq ^{113m}In-DTPA administered in 200 ml of water to image the stomach and proximal intestines and thereby to determine the position of the tablet in the gastro-intestinal tract. Imaging was undertaken using a gamma camera having a 40-cm diameter field of view. Anterior and posterior images were taken over a period of 6 h. The geometric means of the counts from the anterior and posterior images were used to obtain time-activity profiles for the amount of label remaining in the tablet.

The buccal and sublingual tablets were administered to 3 healthy male volunteers. The subjects were seated against the face of the gamma camera. Each subject received the rapidly dissolving tablet (placed in the lower buccal cavity) followed on a second occasion by the sustained release buccal tablet.

Results and Discussion

Oral Sustained Release Tablet

Colour plate I shows a composite picture of some typical images from the radiolabelled tablets following administration. The tablet appears as a white circle. At 15 min and 1 h after dosing the tablet was in the stomach,

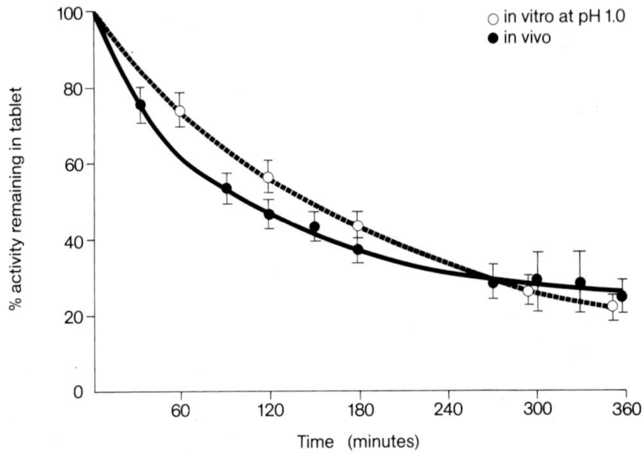

Fig. 1. Comparison of in vitro (○; n = 6) and in vivo (●; n = 4) release of ^{99m}Tc-DTPA from Synchron tablets.

which had been outlined by the ^{113m}In-DTPA. Later images show the tablet in the small intestine. In each of the 4 volunteers the tablet had left the stomach between 1 and 2 h.

Colour plate II shows the appearance of the tablets after different times in the dissolution apparatus. The nature of the swollen gel matrix is clearly seen. The sustained action of the formulation over a period of 6 h or more is achieved by the diffusion of the drug through this gel and the erosion of the gel itself.

The kinetics of drug release [2] conform to those expected for matrix release [13] and a plot of the percentage label remaining in the tablet versus the square root of time gives a linear relationship. A comparison of the in vitro and in vivo release characteristics of the tablets is shown in figure 1. The agreement between the two sets of data is good and it is noted that the release profile in vivo does not change noticeably when the tablets move from stomach to intestine implying that the release characteristics of the matrix is independent of pH. This was confirmed by conducting in vitro release experiments over a range of pH [11].

Buccal Tablets

Figure 2 shows some typical images for the two tablet formulations administered to one of the 3 volunteers. The rapidly dissolving tablet had dis-

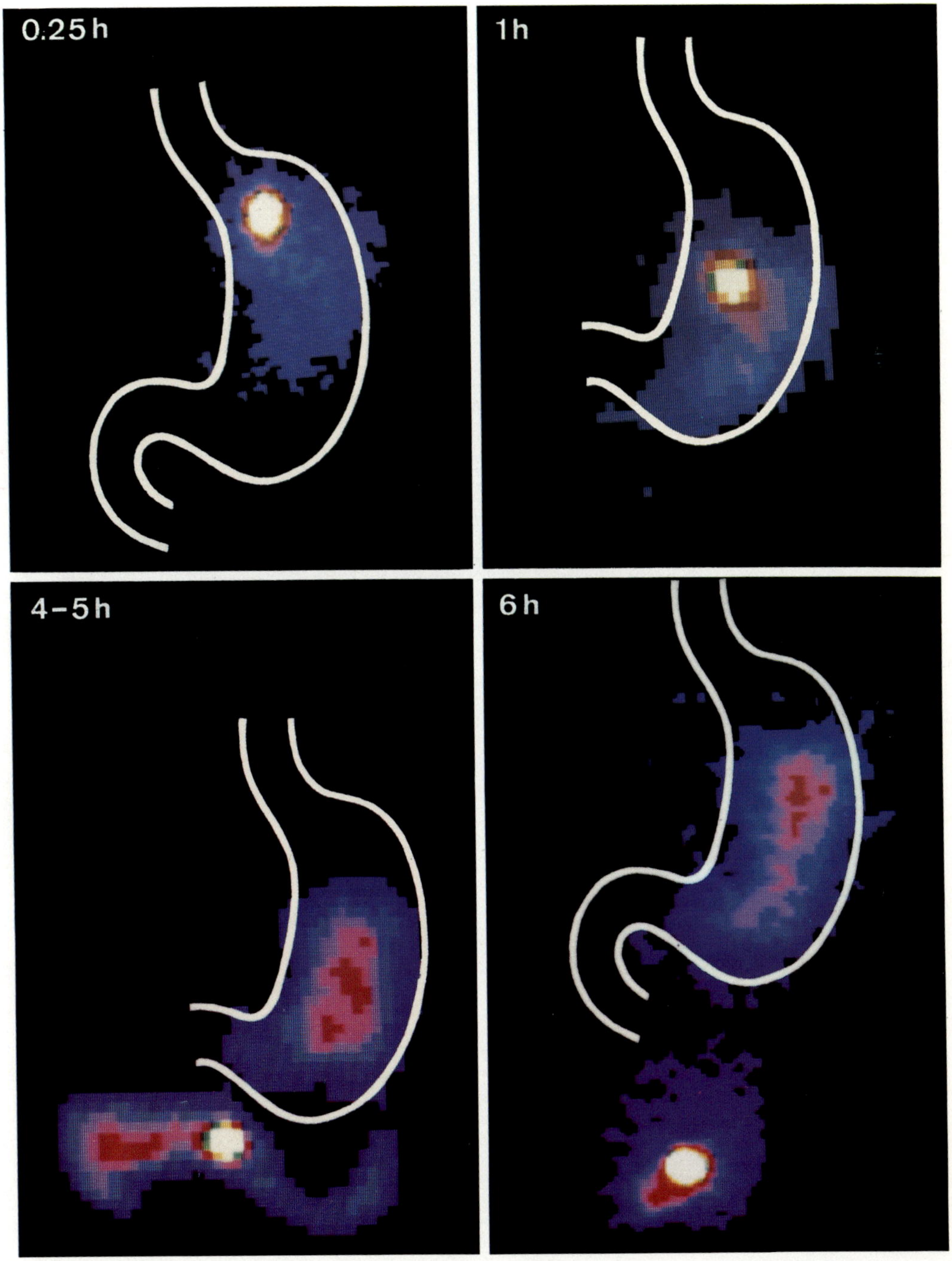

S.S. Davis et al.

Colour Plate I (for legend, see reverse side)

S. Karger, Basel

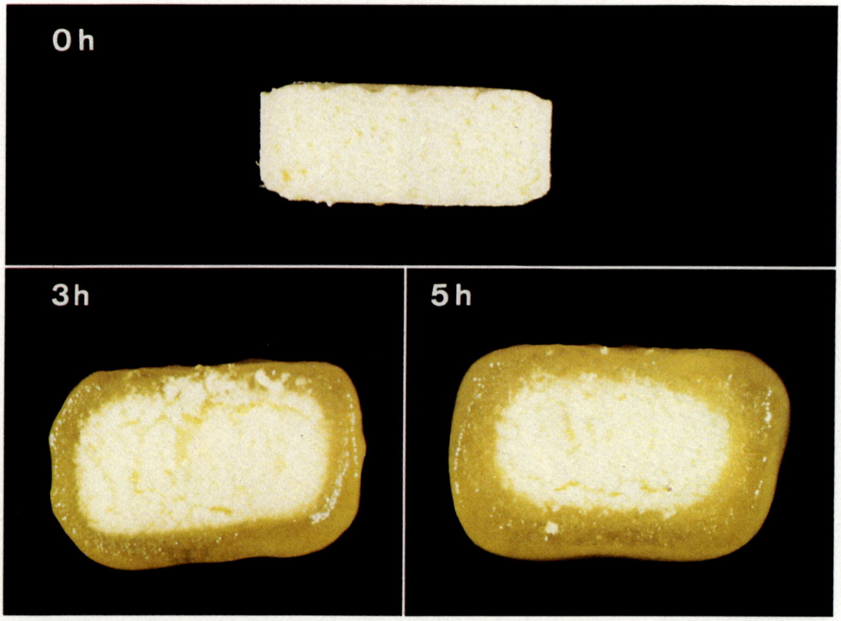

Colour Plate II. Sections of Synchron sustained release tablets after differing periods of time in a dissolution apparatus.

Colour Plate I. Scintigraphic images of oral sustained release tablets in the gastro-intestinal tract at various times after dosing.

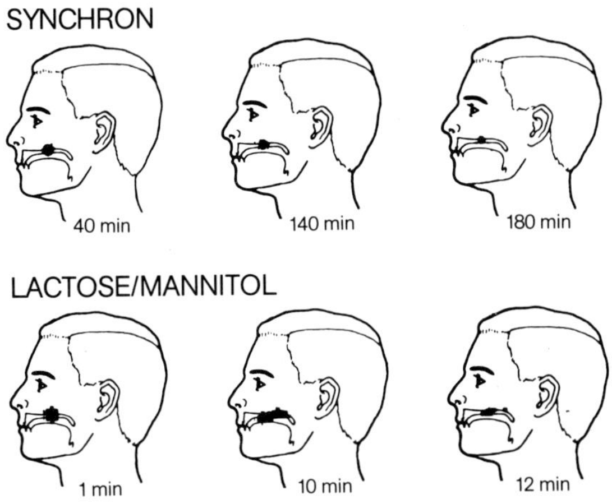

Fig. 2. Scintigraphic images of buccal and sublingual tablets administered to a volunteer.

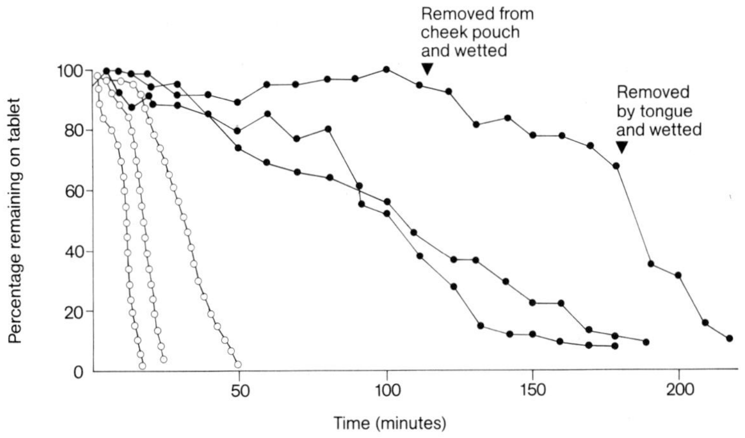

Fig. 3a. Release of ^{99m}Tc-labelled DTPA from mannitol/lactose (○) and Synchron buccal tablets (●).

solved completely after 20 min, while the sustained release Synchron formulation was still releasing the marker after 3 h.

Activity time profiles are given in figure 3 and the difference between the two buccal formulations is clear. The release profiles for the sustained release formulation indicate an approximately linear relationship between the percentage remaining in the tablet and time (zero order release) for 2 of the volunteers. The data for the third volunteer show the importance of position

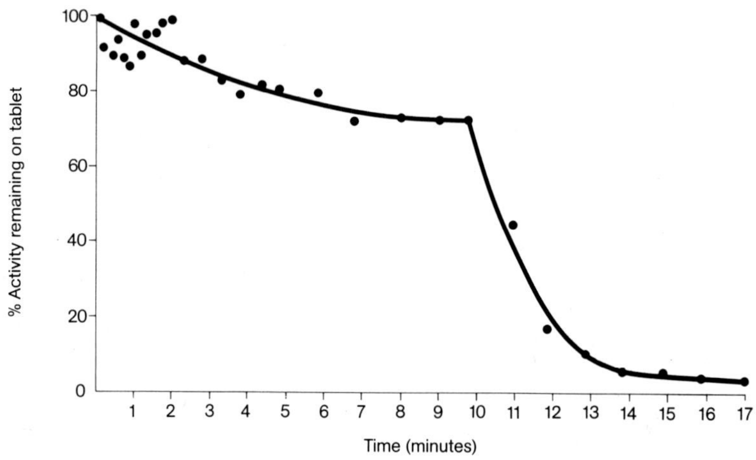

Fig. 3b. Release of ^{99m}Tc-DTPA from sublingual tablet (lactose/mannitol).

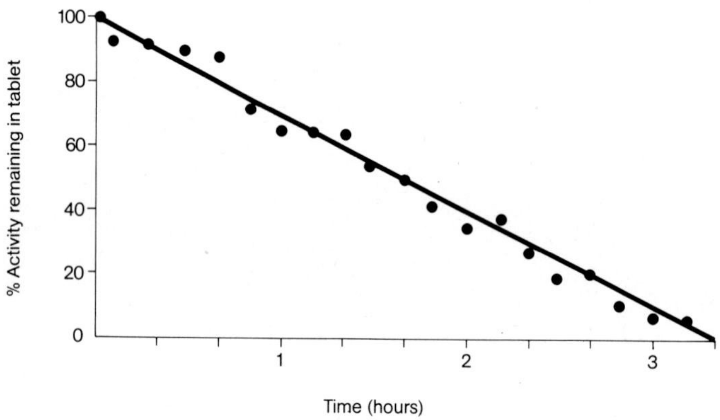

Fig. 3c. Release of ^{99m}Tc-DTPA from Synchron buccal tablets.

of the tablet in the buccal cavity and the effect of wetting and mechanical abrasion. It should also be noted that a volunteer who complained of a dry mouth provided the slowest release for the fast dissolving tablet. The effects of chewing and liquid intake as well as salivary flow are presently under investigation.

A comparison of the release profiles for the orally and buccally administered Synchron systems indicates that the rates and kinetics of release are different. This is due to the effects of the environment but also the amount of the Synchron material incorporated into the tablet. The oral system was made almost totally of Synchron base whereas the buccal system was a 50:50 mixture of Synchron and lactose. It is known that the release characteristics of matrix systems will be influenced by the presence of other excipients, including surface-active agents and diluents [1].

References

1 Lee, V.H.-L.; Robinson, J.R.: Methods to achieve sustained drug delivery. The physical approach, oral and parenteral dosage forms; in Robinson, Sustained and controlled release drug delivery systems, pp. 123–209 (Dekker, New York 1980).

2 Notari, R.E.: Biopharmaceutics and clinical pharmacokinetics; 3rd ed. (Dekker, New York 1980).

3 Ballard, B.E.: An overview of prolonged action drug dosage forms; in Robinson, Sustained and controlled release drug delivery systems, pp. 1–69 (Dekker, New York 1980).

4 Wendkos, M.H.; Meschulam, N.: Comparative effects of placebo and sustained release nitroglycerin in anginal subjects. Preliminary report. J. clin. Pharmacol. J. new Drugs *13:* 160 (1973).

5 Ritschel, W.A.; Clother, R.: Entwicklung einer peroralen Nitroglycerin-Proxyphyllin-Retardform. Arzneimittel-Forsch. *20:* 1180 (1970).

6 Ritschel, W.A.: Influence of formulating factors on the drug safety of time-release nitroglycerin tablets. J. pharm. Sci. *60:* 1683 (1971).

7 Kutscher, A.H.; Zigarelli, E.: A new long-lasting lozenge. Properties and uses. J. oral Ther. Pharm. *4:* 464 (1968).

8 Ganderton, D.: Future developments in tablets and tabletting in good manufacturing practice in tablet manufacture, pp. 113–121 (EFTA, Geneva 1978).

9 Ritschel, W.A.: Peroral solid dosage forms with prolonged action; in Ariens, Drug design, vol. 4 (Academic Press, New York 1973).

10 Daly, P.B.; Davis, S.S.; Frier, M.; Hardy, J.G.; Kennerley, J.W.; Wilson, C.G.: In vitro and in vivo evaluation of a sustained release matrix tablet. J. Pharm. Pharmac. *33:* suppl. 47P (1981).

11 Daly, P.B.; Davis, S.S.; Frier, M.; Hardy, J.G.; Kennerley, J.W.; Wilson, C.G.: Scintigraphic assessment of the in vivo dissolution rate of a sustained release tablet. Int. J. Pharmaceut. *10:* 17–24 (1982).

12 Schor, J.M.: Sustained release therapeutic compositions, United States Patent, 4226849, 1980.

13 Higuchi, T.: Mechanism of sustained action medication. Theoretical analysis of rate of release of solid drugs dispersed in solid matrices. J. pharm. Sci. *52:* 1145–1149 (1963).

S.S. Davis, D. Sc., Department of Pharmacy, University of Nottingham,
Nottingham NG7 2RD (England)

Discussion

Chairman: *H.-L. Fung*

Fung: You presented a very interesting technique in measuring disappearance of drugs from the formulation. I was wondering how you assess the use of ^{99m}Tc in measuring drug release. The polarity of ^{99m}Tc could be substantially different from the drug you may be using and the diffusion coefficient might also be substantially different: how then might you use the radiolabel to relate to actual drug release?

Davis: We have used as our radiolabel ^{99m}Tc and this was incorporated into the model substance DTPA; this is a pentacetic acid material and is highly water-soluble. With a label such as technetium it is possible to bind it into various marker substances, so that one can choose a marker substance that has similarities to the drug molecule that one wishes to study. It is extremely difficult with the technique of gamma scintigraphy to incorporate a gamma label into a drug molecule. So we have to use a model substance that we believe is similar to our drug molecule. Before we started the studies in man we compared using dissolution tests the release of our technetium labelled chelate and drug substances, to make sure we were looking at the same sort of process. We chose the DTPA material because it is not absorbed from the gastro-intestinal tract, and was ideal for our purposes in studying where was the tablet and then how much of our marker had been released from the formulation.

Fung: I may also add, as most of you are aware of from Dr. *Abrams'* talk, that Prof. *Needleman* had shown that there is a substantial first-pass metabolism of these nitrates, and we have shown recently in animal studies that this first-pass metabolism can be substantially saturated. I think that it was unfortunate, in a way, that Prof. *Needleman* had done this a long time ago using very low doses of nitroglycerin. We could, by increasing the doses of nitroglycerin in animals, show substantial bioavailability after oral administration because the first-pass metabolism can be saturated. The reason I mention this is that in the design of these sustained release systems, it becomes extremely important to program the correct rate of delivery, because if you program the rate in too slow a manner for input into the gastro-intestinal tract, the first-pass metabolism becomes very, very extensive. So in designing sustained release oral systems of nitrates, it would almost be working at cross-purposes in that by sustaining the delivery, you're inputting the drug at a very slow rate and, with this slow delivery the first-pass metabolism can become very substantial. The bioavailability can then be substantially decreased for this particular reason. In my mind, at this point, it becomes very critical to understand the concentration versus first-pass relationship if one were to rationally design oral sustained release systems of organic nitrates.

Davis: I would like to add to that. With a matrix system, such as the Synchron system, one can adjust the amount of the Synchron material, the amount of additives, give the sort of release rate that one wants so as to avoid the first-pass effect. Propranolol is another drug that has considerable first-pass metabolism, but is marketed as a sustained release pellet system.

Schor: What you say is correct. We did take that into account when we designed the rates in these tablets. We felt that the absolute amount exposed to the liver per hour was the governing factor, if you could saturate the liver by keeping the amount released above a certain level, then you could get material into the circulation.

Reichek: I wonder whether it might not be important to include vasoactivation; we were specifically interested in the test tablet for the oral route. It wasn't clear to me whether you did that, since nitroglycerin is a vasoactive substance. One could readily imagine that it might, in fact, alter the gastro-intestinal physiology and affect the dissolution of the tablet itself.

Davis: Yes, indeed. The results I've shown are the first set of experiments we've done on the oral and buccal formulations. We are aware that the pharmacological agent, whether it be nitroglycerin or any other pharmacological agent, may well have an effect. For example, in the buccal study we want to look at the effect of nitroglycerin on saliva flow. We should be able to study these effects with our technique of scintigraphy.

Bussmann: We had a few patients who dissolved the buccal tablets within 10 min. Others had their tablets for longer times – 1 or 2 h. You showed data on 2–3 h. Did you ever experience a patient that could dissolve the buccal tablets within 10 min?

Davis: We found, with volunteers who had dry mouths, that we got a very slow release. But in no occasion did we find a very rapid release with these formulations. 10 min sounds very quick for the Synchron system. A much slower release than that would be expected. I have a feeling that the volunteer or patient was doing something unusual with the tablet. For example moving it around the mouth, rather than letting it remain stationary in the buccal cavity.

Schor: In line with that, we set up experiments where we asked people to move the tablets with their tongue every few minutes between the four pouches and we were able to halve the dissolution time to about 45 min. As a control we asked them to keep the tablet in one place throughout the experiment. This served as a baseline and we found that there was no dissolution of the tablet before at least 1.5 h of residence time in the buccal pouch had passed.

Adv. Pharmacother., vol. 1, pp. 26–34 (Karger, Basel 1982)

Factors Affecting the Determination and Interpretation of Nitroglycerin Pharmacokinetics

H.-L. Fung

Department of Pharmaceutics, School of Pharmacy,
State University of New York at Buffalo, Buffalo, N.Y., USA

Research on nitroglycerin has experienced a tremendous upsurge in recent years because of its expanded clinical use in patients after acute myocardial infarction [1], congestive heart failure [2] and unstable angina [3]. Newer modes of administration of this drug have also become more popular: these include (1) continuous intravenous infusion for the management of acutely ill patients, and (2) sustained-release formulations for prolonging the beneficial effects of nitroglycerin. The latter formulations have been prepared for buccal, oral, transdermal or rectal [4] delivery. The availability of analytical methods capable of detecting trace levels of nitroglycerin in biological fluids have made the assessment of these different formulations in humans feasible.

Pharmacokinetic studies of nitroglycerin in humans were made possible by the pioneering efforts of *Rosseel and Bogaert* [5] who developed the first workable assay method for determining nitroglycerin in plasma. Subsequently, several research groups [6–8] have worked to modify this method resulting in improvements in sensitivity and ease of operation. A summary of the various gas chromatographic methods has been presented elsewhere [9].

Pharmacokinetic studies of nitroglycerin are comparatively more difficult to conduct than those of many other drugs because of the rather unique combination of its pharmacokinetic and physicochemical properties. Nitroglycerin is rapidly cleared from blood after therapeutic doses. Therefore, blood or plasma nitroglycerin concentrations during therapy are typically less than 5 ng/ml. Assay of these low concentrations is further complicated by the high volatility, high adsorptivity to plastic and chemical instability of this drug. Numerous precautions need to be taken to assure accurate and reproducible determination of nitroglycerin concentrations in biological fluids.

Factors Affecting the Determination of Nitroglycerin in Plasma

The basic extraction and gas chromatographic procedures used at Buffalo for the determination of plasma nitroglycerin have been outlined previously [6]. Here, I shall only go into additional comments on the assay and some of the modifications that we have made since its publication.

A major problem of the nitroglycerin assay that needs to be prevented is contamination, either from atmospheric nitroglycerin which escapes into the laboratory air-space or from non-specific interference. Because of the high volatility of nitroglycerin and the very small amounts of it which eventually end up in the chromatograph (typically around 5–50 pg on column), great care must be taken not to contaminate the assay laboratory, glassware, solvent, evaporation system, etc. with the drug. Handling of bulk powders or bulk solutions, even though they may contain milligram quantities of nitroglycerin, must be carried out away from the assay laboratory and systems. One soon learns from painful experience, as we have done in our earlier years of the assay, that lack of quarantine of the assay from even what might normally be considered minute quantities of nitroglycerin might spell long hours and days of unfruitful assays, loss of samples, and the necessity of arduous decontamination efforts.

The maintenance of 'super-cleaned' glassware, according to our experience, is another important criterion for successful execution of the nitroglycerin assay. In our laboratory, all glassware is subjected to a cleaning and silanization procedure as described below: the glassware is soaked in a chromic/sulfuric acid mixture overnight, then rinsed thoroughly with distilled water and dried thoroughly in a hot-air oven. Silanization is carried out by soaking the glassware in a 10% solution of dimethyldichlorosilane in toluene for at least 30 min, then rinsing sequentially with toluene, a 1:1 mixture of toluene and methanol, reagent-grade methanol and finally pesticide-grade methanol. The treated glassware is then dried in a hot-air oven and kept in a covered container before use.

In our published procedure [6], we have recommended multiple extraction of plasma with hexane to effect quantitative recovery of nitroglycerin. This extraction procedure may be considered cumbersome, although, in experienced hands, it is not (it does require, however, rather strong fingers

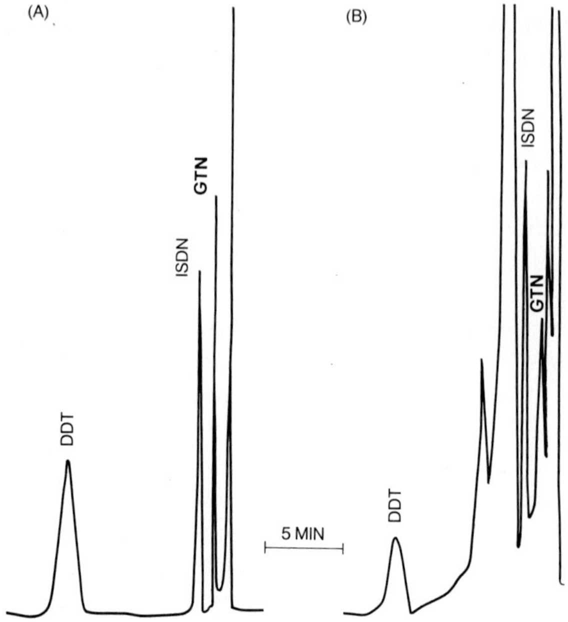

Fig. 1. Chromatograms of an external standard solution (A) and a plasma sample (B) containing 2.0 ng/ml of nitroglycerin and 8.0 ng/ml of isosorbide dinitrate. Both drugs were administered to the patient.

and wrist if high productivity is desired!). This concern, however, is not as serious as the occurrence of possible operator-dependent recovery of nitroglycerin as obtained from different analysts, since the degree of mixing in each extraction step cannot be rigorously standardized. We have now modified the extraction step as follows: plasma samples (100–500 μl) are shaken twice with 2 ml of pesticide-grade hexane, 15 min each time; the organic phases are combined and evaporated to 20–50 μl under nitrogen before injection into the chromatograph. This modification does not affect the recovery of nitroglycerin but has led to better reproducibility.

The ideal internal standard to be used for assay of samples from experimental pharmacokinetic studies is isosorbide dinitrate. However, for clinical samples in which the concomitant presence of nitroglycerin and isosorbide dinitrate is either known or suspected, use of this internal standard is not possible. We have found that the pesticide DDT is useful as an alternate internal standard, particularly when the concentration of nitroglycerin in plasma is below 2 ng/ml. In these samples, non-specific interference sometimes becomes significant around the isosorbide dinitrate peak, whereas it is seldom so around the DDT peak. We routinely check the plasma samples for DDT blanks and we have found that environmentally acquired DDT concentrations in plasma are insignificant compared to what is added for assay. Figure 1 shows the chromatographic characteristics of nitroglycerin, isosorbide dinitrate and DDT in a standard (panel a) and from a plasma sample (panel b).

In many of our collaborative studies which involve trans-continental or inter-continental shipment of samples, we include another standardization procedure to monitor the handling and degradation of these samples during transit. For each patient, a blank blood sample (10 ml) is collected before the initiation of the study, centrifuged to separate plasma and divided into 5–1 ml plasma aliquots. To four of these samples are added 25 μl of various accurate solutions of nitroglycerin such that the final plasma samples contain 0.5, 1, 2 and 5 ng/ml of nitroglycerin. These 'standards' are then processed and stored in the same manner as the unknown samples before and during shipment. The recovery determined from these 'standards' will be used as a correction factor for each patient.

Factors Affecting the Interpretation of Nitroglycerin Pharmacokinetics

Despite the great care that has been taken in the assay of samples, the plasma concentrations so determined still present considerable difficulty for pharmacokinetic interpretation. A recent study which examines the kinetics of nitroglycerin in normal subjects after intravenous infusion [10] shows nitroglycerin to possess the following pharmacokinetic properties: (1) intra- and inter-subject variability in nitroglycerin plasma kinetics is substantial, this may, in part, be due to (2) the very large apparent plasma clearance, 0.3 to 1 liter/min/kg, of the drug, (3) the plasma half-life is very short (ca 3 min) and, (4) the apparent volume of distribution is large, at about 3 liters/kg, suggesting that plasma drug can only account for only about 1% of the total drug in the body. Table I shows the detailed pharmacokinetics of nitroglycerin in the subjects studied. Since about 99% of the total body load in nitroglycerin is outside the plasma compartment, minor fluctuations in drug distribution and/or binding in this large extra-plasma compartment, which can be produced by a number of internal or external stimuli, could cause a relatively large change in the plasma concentrations, and hence, in the calculated pharmacokinetic parameters. In fact, in 2 of the subjects studied, plasma nitroglyc-

Table I. Pharmacokinetic data obtained after intravenous nitroglycerin infusion in normal subjects. From McNiff et al. [10]

Subject	Infusion rate µg/min	Dose µg	K min^{-1}	$t_{1/2}$ min	V_d l/kg	$Cl_s = \frac{D}{AUC}$ l/min/kg	$Cl^* = \frac{k_o}{C_{32}}$ l/min/kg	Apparent steady state achieved
5B	18.9	605	0.52	1.3	1.7	0.31 (29.8)	0.33	yes
7	16.4	524	0.21	3.3	2.4	0.49 (37.7)	0.43	yes
8	16.5	527	0.19	3.7	2.9	0.54 (31.3)	0.57	yes
3	18.6	596	0.25	2.8	4.1	1.02 (73.4)	0.67	no
4	15.5	496	0.18	3.8	5.2	0.94 (60.2)	0.66	no
5A	16.6	531	0.31	2.2	2.4	0.74 (71.0)	0.47	no
9	18.6	598	0.31	2.2	4.1	1.03 (78.3)	0.90	no
6	18.2	584	–	–	–	–	–	–
10	21.5	688	–	–	–	–	–	–
Mean	17.9	573	0.28	2.8	3.3	0.72 (54.5)	0.58	–
± SD	1.8	59	0.12	0.9	1.2	0.28 (21.1)	0.19	–

Numbers in parentheses represent total body clearance (Cl_s × body weight), l/min. K = Apparent elimination constant; $t_{1/2}$ = plasma half-life; V_d = apparent volume of distribution; Cl_s = apparent systemic clearance; D = dose; AUC = area under the plasma concentration vs time curve; k_o = infusion rate; C_{32} = nitroglycerin concentration in plasma at 32 min, end of infusion.

erin concentrations were oscillating to such an extent that pharmacokinetic analysis could not be performed. In some subjects, 'steady-state' concentrations were not observed, contrary to expectation because of its short half-life, and a rebound in plasma concentrations during the post-infusion phase was evident. For detailed discussion, the reader is referred to the original manuscript [10].

A question in nitroglycerin kinetics that has so far not been addressed is whether blood or plasma concentration is more pertinent. If red blood cells (RBC) accumulate nitroglycerin significantly and RBC and plasma drug did not equilibrate rapidly, then plasma kinetics may only be a partial picture. We have recently conducted a study [11] in which we showed, in both human and rat blood, that RBC and plasma nitroglycerin are rapidly equilibrating and that the rates of decline of nitroglycerin in equilibrating RBC and plasma are similar. Interestingly, the RBC/plasma nitroglycerin concentration ratio is 0.4 ± 0.3 (mean ± SD) in human blood, in contrast to a ratio of 2.6 ± 1.1 (mean ± SD) in rat blood. Using an approximate value of 0.45 as hematocrit, blood nitroglycerin concentration can be estimated to be 0.73 and 1.72 times that in plasma, for human and the rat, respectively.

Another important question in the interpretation of nitroglycerin kinetics relates to the site of sampling of nitroglycerin in the vasculature. Several groups of workers [12–14] showed that systemic nitroglycerin concentration can be highly dependent on the site of blood withdrawal. We recently carried out a study in dogs to examine this question. We found [15] that the arterial plasma clearance of nitroglycerin to be approximately 2.7 times slower than venous clearance. These results supported a model of nitroglycerin clearance which involves contribution from blood vessel wall transport and/or metabolism [16]. The rates of these processes in the arterial and venous vasculatures may be substantially different.

Although the mechanistic interpretation of nitroglycerin kinetics may be difficult, for the reasons indicated above, the use of nitroglycerin plasma concentrations in comparing the systemic availability of different pharmaceutical dosage forms is still feasible. If great care is taken to standardize experimental procedures in identical fashion when different dosage forms are tested, and sensitive and reproducible assay procedures are used, comparison of plasma concentrations and the pharmacokinetic estimates can provide useful information relating to the absorption characteristics of these products.

Acknowledgements

This work was supported in part by NIH Grants HL22273 and GM20852. The contributions from my co-workers (identified in the references) are gratefully acknowledged. The excellent technical assistance from *D. Ruggirello, A. Poliszczuk* and *J. Dolce* is appreciated.

References

1 Armstrong, P.W.; Walker, D.C.; Burton, J.R.; Parker, J.O.: Vasodilator therapy in acute myocardial infarction. A comparison of sodium nitroprusside and nitroglycerin. Circulation *52:* 1118 (1975).

2 Mikulic, E.; Franciosa, J.A.; Cohn, J.N.: Comparative hemodynamic effects of chewable isosorbide dinitrate and nitroglycerin in patients with congestive heart failure. Circulation *52:* 477 (1975).

3 Oliva, P.B.; Plots, D.E.; Pluss, R.G.: Coronary arterial spasm in Prinzmetal angina. New Engl. J. Med. *288:* 745 (1973).

4 Kamiya, A.; Ogata, H.; Fung, H.-L.: Rectal absorption of nitroglycerin in the rat: avoidance of first-pass metabolism as a function of rectal length exposure. J. pharm. Sci. (in press, 1982).

5 Rosseel, M.T.; Bogaert, M.G.: GLC determination of nitroglycerin and isosorbide dinitrate in human plasma. J. pharm. Sci. *62:* 754 (1973).

6 Yap, S.K.; McNiff, E.F.; Fung, H.-L.: An improved GLC assay for the determination of nitroglycerin in plasma. J. pharm. Sci. *67:* 682 (1978).

7 Wei, J.Y.; Reid, P.R.: Quantitative determination of trinitroglycerin in human plasma. Circulation *59:* 588 (1979).

8 Armstrong, P.W.; Armstrong, J.A.; Marks, G.S.: Blood levels after sublingual nitroglycerin. Circulation *59:* 585 (1979).

9 McNiff, E.F.; Yap, P.S.K.; Fung, H.-L.: Nitroglycerin; in Florey, Analytical profiles of drug substances, vol. 9 (Academic Press, New York 1980).

10 McNiff, E.F.; Yacobi, A.; Young-Chang, F.M.; Golden, L.H.; Goldfarb, A.; Fung, H.-L.: Pharmacokinetics of nitroglycerin after intravenous infusion in normal subjects. J. pharm. Sci. *70:* 1054 (1981).

11 Kamiya, A.; Schmitt, T.; Fung, H.-L.: Unpublished data.

12 Brymer, J.F.; Stetson, P.L.; Walton, J.A., Jr.; Lucchesi, B.; Pitt, B.: Correlation of hemodynamic effects and plasma levels of nitroglycerin. Clin. Res. *27:* 229A (1979).

13 Armstrong, P.W.; Armstrong, J.A.; Marks, G.S.: Plasma nitroglycerin gradient during intravenous infusion in man. Circulation *62:* 326 (1980).

14 Hill, A.B.; Bowley, C.J.; Nahrwold, M.L.; Knight, P.R.; Kirsh, M.M.; Denlinger, J.K.: Intranasal administration of nitroglycerin. Anesthesiology *54:* 346 (1981).

15 Fung, H.-L.; McNiff, E.F.; Lai, C.M.; Look, Z.M.; Yacobi, A.: Unpublished data.

16 Kamiya, A.; Fung, H.-L.: Abstract of paper 1087. Disposition of nitroglycerin in rat plasma and selected blood vessels. 8th Int. Congr. of Pharmacology, Tokyo 1981.

H.-L. Fung, PhD, Department of Pharmaceutics, School of Pharmacy,
State University of New York at Buffalo, Buffalo, NY 14260 (USA)

Discussion

Chairman: *W.-D. Bussmann*

Woodcock: I found your paper very interesting. I think you have gone to the essence of the pharmacokinetic problem with nitroglycerin. You told us that only 1% of the drug could be found in the blood or plasma, and that the rest of the drug was found in the tissues. I would like to ask you if you have measured the half-life of nitroglycerin in blood vessels, since this may give us an indication of the true bioavailability and also of the concentrations at the site of action?

Fung: Yes. We have done some studies in animals that investigate the pharmacokinetics of nitroglycerin in blood vessels. I too view that in order to understand the pharmacology of tolerance, we cannot just look at plasmakinetics as the only component. I believe that vessel kinetics are more important. We have finished a study which shows that blood vessel kinetics of nitroglycerin are considerably slower than that of nitroglycerin – in rats. This occurs both in the venous vessels as well as in the arterial vessels. The approximate half-life difference in the rat is about two times to three times, that is, the half-life of nitroglycerin in blood vessels is two or three times longer than that of plasma half-life. This is consistent with the general observation, I believe, that the pharmacodynamics of nitroglycerin have a longer half-life than that of plasma half-life. I believe the blood vessel kinetics are a very important component if we were to understand the duration of action, and the tolerance behavior, which are associated with these organic nitrates.

Windorfer: When we started our studies with the determination of nitroglycerin, the preparation was done in the same manner as in your laboratory with silver nitrate. But later we saw that it wasn't necessary to take silver nitrate. When you froze the sample at once after taking it at −20 °C then we found that the sample remained stable for some weeks, but then it is not allowed to interrupt the freezing. But another problem that we realized and also found in the literature, was the adsorption of nitroglycerin to some plastic material. We found that the adsorption of GTN to plastic material occurred after a short time, for example after half an hour. Therefore, we think it is necessary to fill the sample directly after blood-taking into a silanized glass.

Fung: I think the silver nitrate addition is historic for us. We have done the recovery study with silver nitrate and it was too late for us to change when we did the animal and clinical experiments. Other people have also related that silver nitrate may not be necessary. We found that it somehow seemed to increase the recovery slightly. Therefore, we have stuck with it. I tend to agree with you that the addition of silver nitrate may not be crucial. The other question relating to plastic is a very important one because there are many data that have suggested that i.v. infusion using plastic bags and delivery tubes showed substantial adsorption. Therefore, the data that are generated could be highly unreliable in terms of the dose administered. Not only is it a pharmaceutical problem, it is a problem of interpreting clinical literature. What really is the dose that was given? Some of you may know that in the United States there are some companies that are poised to market non-adsorbing tubing delivery sets for nitroglycerin. We found in terms of the analysis that soft plastics, for example polyvinylchloride, adsorbed nitroglycerin. High-density polyethylene seems to be a plastic that had no adsorptive properties, so during our infusion, if we were to use high-density polyethylene, it seemed to be OK. But we, like you, rather than reinventing the wheel and doing something that we're not quite sure of, have stuck with glass and silanized glass all the time. Those of you who might be involved with the assay know that the cleanliness of the glassware and the silanization of glassware is very important, and we silanize everything in sight that we use. This represents tremendous organic solvent waste, but I think that it is important for the good of the assay.

Békés: Is it possible to neglect the so-called 'natural nitro elements' of the body in such a fine determination as yours?

Fung: Is it possible to neglect the natural nitro bodies? Well, what we usually do is obviously take blank samples during the studies. We not only take blank samples for determination of nitroglycerin levels, but we also determine the internal standard level because we are adding also very small amounts of internal standards. So in almost all of our samples we first run the blank without adding anything to get a handle on it. We generally found that the apparent endogenous concentration of nitroglycerin is quite small. They are generally in the range of maybe 0.1–0.2 ng/ml. Therefore, if we want to do kinetics down to 0.1–0.5 ng/ml, it is a very difficult process. We really have to have everything superclean. The persons have to almost be washed clean of nitroglycerin completely before we do it.

Bussmann: You said that nitroglycerin goes into the tissue, into the veins, into the arteries, what kind of other tissues are there? We saw, as you said, following i.v. nitroglycerin, the hemodynamic effect takes 2–4 h to go back to the control level.

Fung: It's not only the vessels. We have done isolated perfused vessels studies and we found that the vessels take up nitroglycerin substantially, but they're also very permeable to nitroglycerin. So if you were to perfuse a vessel, more than 80% of the drug goes into the extravascular space. So I would say, with the interesting solubility characteristic of nitroglycerin, that it is equally soluble or equally insoluble in water and organic solvents – that it is likely to be distributed all over. Interestingly enough, there has never been a study, as far as I know, that looked at the radiography of nitroglycerin to determine how and where the drug is distributed in different tissue space. We intend to see whether we have enough ^{14}C-nitroglycerin to do that experiment.

Bussmann: After oral nitroglycerin very low plasma levels are present. It may be that during the passage through the intestines a large tissue can be filled up with nitroglycerin. May this be the cause for low plasma levels, independent of the first-pass problem?

Fung: Yes, I think it is possible. I think there was some data which shows that after oral administration of nitroglycerin in oil, there is a large concentration of radioactivity that is left in the intestine for a long period of time. One doesn't know whether the particular dosage form, that is, the oil, had contributed to it. Yes, I think the uptake of nitroglycerin by tissues during transit is a very important phenomenon because the drug seems to have a great affinity for tissue. The hypothesis that the orally acting nitroglycerin is made somewhat ineffective through first-pass metabolism as well as tissue uptake yielding non-productive metabolite is certainly a feasible one.

Adv. Pharmacother., vol. 1, pp. 35–43 (Karger, Basel 1982)

Bioavailability of Controlled Release Buccal and Oral Nitroglycerin by Digital Plethysmography

Randall J. Erb

Pharmadynamics Research, Inc., West Lafayette, Ind., USA

Background

In 1973, an FDA-sponsored project at Purdue University [1] began investigating the use of cardiovascular pharmacological response measure as direct indicators of the physiological vasodilator activity which underlies the clinical response to organic nitrate antianginal drugs. 'This work clearly indicates that physiological response methodology can provide reliable, sensitive, convenient, and meaningful measures of the drug's bioavailability…' [2]. The digital plethysmographic (DPG) parameter, diastolic amplitude response, was utilized to demonstrate the bioavailability of oral and buccal nitroglycerin dosage forms.

Materials and Methods

Two studies were untertaken to investigate oral and buccal sustained action dosage forms following FDA guidelines for DPG studies [3]:

2.6-mg oral Synchron GTN tablet (lot 58467)
6.5-mg oral Synchron GTN tablet (lots 4-7-77 and 10515)
10.0-mg oral Synchron GTN tablet (lot 11-8-77)
1.0-mg buccal Synchron GTN tablet (lot 10779)
2.5-mg buccal Synchron GTN tablet (lot 605-5-80)
5.0-mg buccal Synchron GTN tablet (lot 4-6-77)

Prior to initiation, protocols and informed consent forms were reviewed and approved by an Institutional Review Board. Each subject signed an informed consent form which complied with HEW guidelines regarding consent forms for human drug studies.

Male volunteers, 18–35 years old, stable, responsible, and cooperative were recruited. Subjects were healthy, free of allergies and were within ± 10% of the Desirable Weights of Adults (Statist. Bull Metrop. Life Insurance Co., 40, Nov.–Dec., 1959).

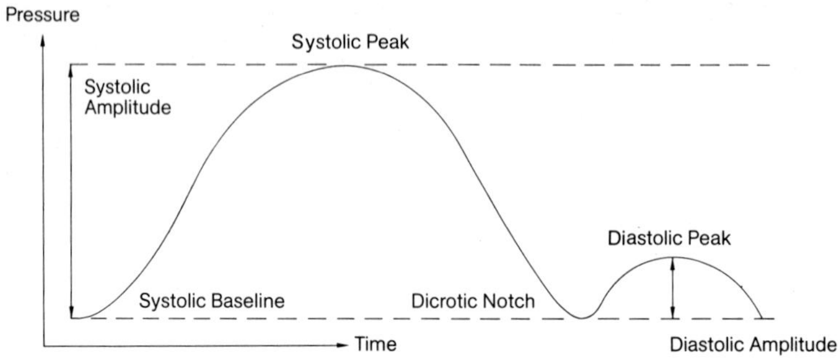

Fig. 1. Characteristics of a DPG wave.

Each subject passed a physical examination including laboratory testing covering: (a) hematology: hemoglobin, hematocrit, WBC differential, especially granulocytes; (b) blood chemistry: BUN, serum alkaline phosphatase, serum bilirubin and SGOT; (c) urinanalysis: specific gravity, protein, glucose, occult blood, acetone and a microscopic examination; (d) 12-lead electrocardiogram and exercise tolerance test.

The studies were designed as complete double-blind crossovers. Each study contained a placebo and 0.6-mg sublingual nitroglycerin tablet dose for internal references.

The subject would recline in a hospital bed at a 30° angle. A DPG transducer was secured to the middle finger of the subject's left hand, but not to the extent that the circulation at the finger-tip was significantly influenced. A Harvard Apparatus 361 pulse transducer was employed for his measurement. The transducer was connected to an AC/DC input coupler in a Beckman Model 511A Dynograph®. The DPG signal was then amplified to obtain an optimal waveform. The output from the Dynograph was connected to the input of a Hewlett-Packard 396A Instrumentation tape recorder through appropriate switching circuitry. Three Beckmann® electrocardiogram (ECG) electrodes were secured to the subject in a lead I configuration and the ECG was recorded in the same manner as the DPG.

Once the equipment was calibrated and the subject's DPG signals were checked, predrug readings were initiated. Seven predrug readings were taken, the last six of which were analyzed and averaged as the predrug baseline for the DPG responses.

The time at which each subject received the drug was considered postdrug time 0. After dosing, DPG readings were taken at the following intervals: 3, 6, 9, 12, 15, 18, 21, 24, 27, 30, 36, 42, 48, 54, 60, 75, 90, 105, 120, 135, 150, 165, 180, 195, 210, 225, 240, lunch break, 270, 285, 300, 315, 330, 345, 360, 375, 390, 405, 420, 435, 450, 465, and 480 min. When the subjects received the sublingual dose, data were collected only up to 300 min postdrug.

Each data interval consisted of a 10- to 12-second period during which the subject held his breath while his DPG signal was recorded on electromagnetic tape. A paper strip chart record of the DPG signal was also obtained during this period. The strip chart was run at a rate of 10 mm/s.

The data were analyzed using a Rockland 452 filter and a Hewlett Packard 2100S microprogrammable systems computer, including a 5466 analog-to-digital converter and a 5451B Fourier analyzer.

The diastolic amplitude response intensity values (DPG-DA) data consisted of three parameters combined. The diastolic amplitude itself is the distance from the lowest point in the dicrotic notch to the maximum of the diastolic peak (fig. 1). The average value of predrug diastolic amplitude was substracted from the average diastolic amplitude for each postdrug data interval. This value was then divided by the predrug systolic amplitude average (systolic peak-systolic baseline value), i.e.

$$\text{diastolic amplitude response intensity} = \frac{\text{postdrug diastolic amplitude average at time t} - \text{predrug diastolic amplitude average}}{\text{predrug systolic amplitude average}}.$$

The numerical values of these parameters were obtained by computer processing and the DPG-DA intensity values and areas under the response intensity curves for various time intervals were obtained. Areas under the curves (AUCs) were calculated by the trapezoidal rule. Statistical analysis was then performed on all AUC value differences of each test drug from placebo using paired t-tests. The AUC calculations and paired t-test comparisons were performed by an in-house program, ANLYSN.

Results and Discussion

In the first study, 6.5 and 10 mg oral Synchron nitroglycerin (GTN) controlled release (CR) dosage forms were tested using 12 subjects. The placebo-corrected results are shown in figure 2. The sublingual GTN response is characteristic of most sublingual responses, peaking at 3 min and lasting 30–60 min. The 6.5-mg oral Synchron GTN dose reaches a plateau at about 30 min and lasts 5 h (i.e. it demonstrates statistically significant activity, alpha = 0.05, compared to placebo).

In a later study (fig. 3), a 6.5-mg oral Synchron GTN dose was tested in 20 subjects. The results were similar to the first study. This is seen in figures 4 and 5. As can be seen in figure 5, the total response ellicited over a 7.5-hour period for the dosage forms was very nearly the same.

The first study also tested a 10-mg oral Synchron GTN form (fig. 6). Compared to the 6.5-mg dose, 10 mg produced only a slightly larger DPG response. This is undoubtedly due to the near saturation of the DPG response in this group of normal subjects. The controlled release properties of the dosage form are again apparent from the plateau in activity which exists for nearly 5 h after the peak effect at 24 min.

A 2.6-mg oral Synchron GTN CR dosage form was tested (fig. 7). It produced observable activity for 7 h and was statistically significant from placebo for 4 h. Although lower, its activity profile was generally the same as the 6.5- and 10-mg doses.

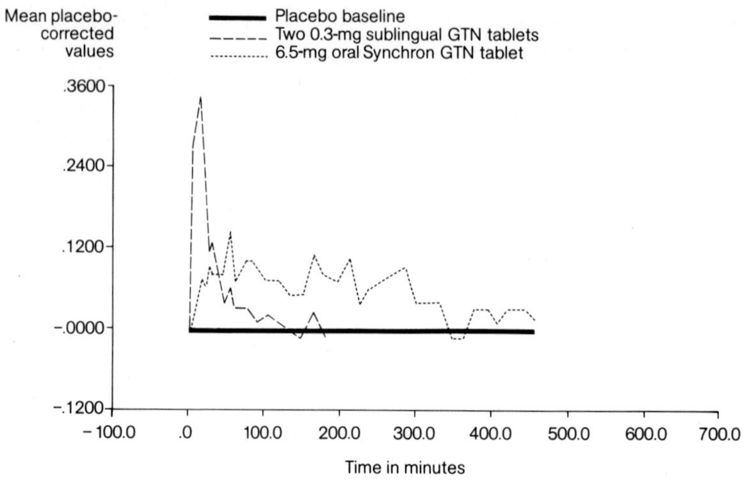

Fig. 2. Mean placebo-corrected DPG response for 0.6-mg sublingual and 6.5-mg oral Synchron GTN (lot 4-7-77).

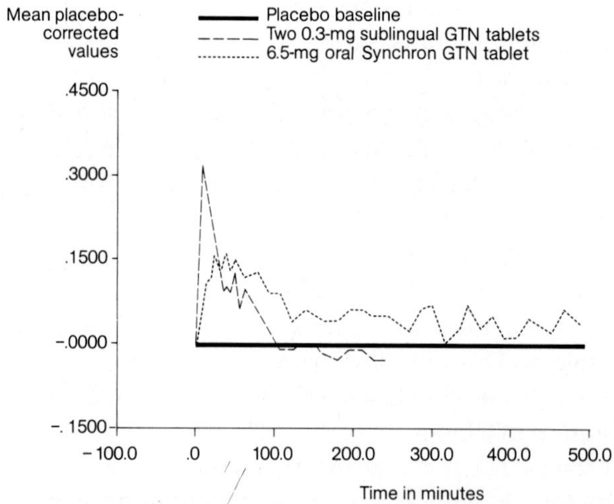

Fig. 3. Mean placebo-corrected DPG response for 0.6-mg sublingual GTN and 6.5-mg oral Synchron GTN (lot 10515).

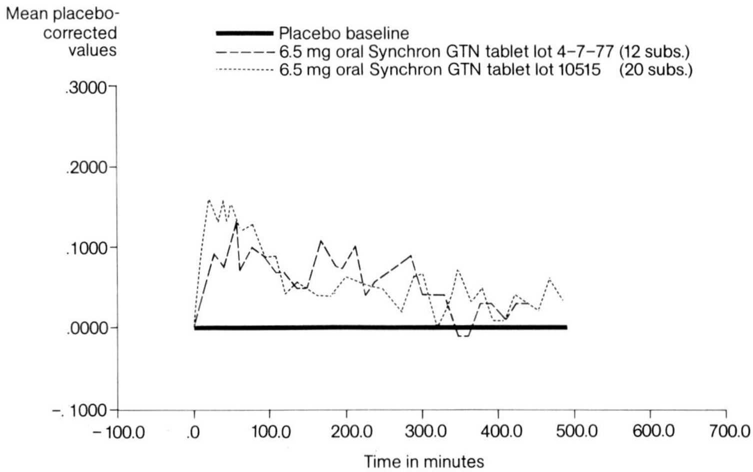

Fig. 4. A mean placebo-corrected DPG response comparison of 2 different lots of 6.5-mg oral Synchron GTN-controlled release tablets administered to two groups of subjects on different occasions.

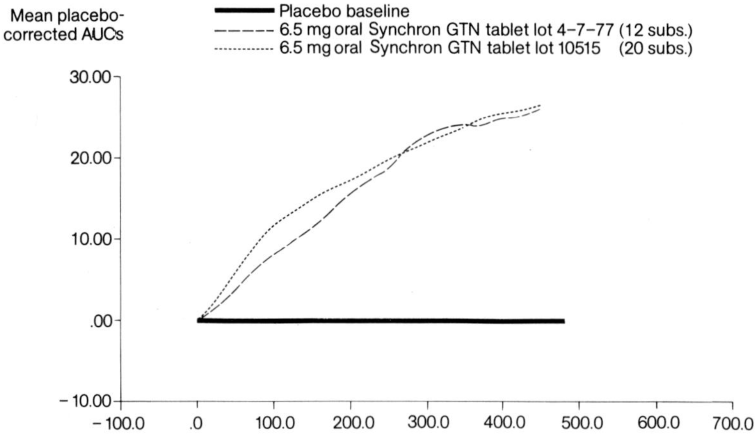

Fig. 5. Cumulative AUC for figure 4 comparing 2 different lots of 6.5-mg oral Synchron GTN-controlled release tablets administered to two subject groups.

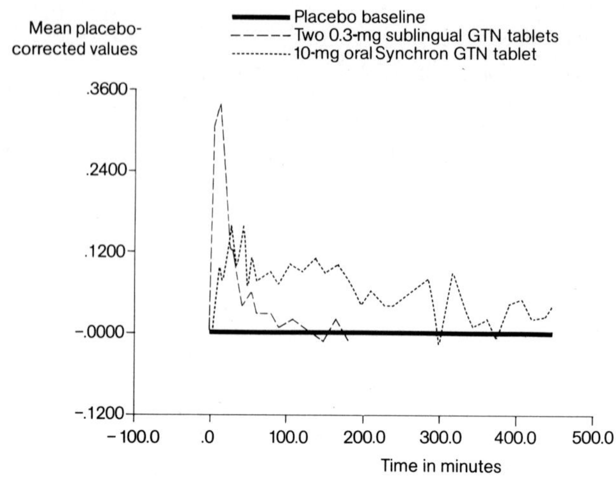

Fig. 6. Mean placebo-corrected DPG response for 0.6-mg sublingual GTN tablets and a 10-mg oral Synchron GTN CR formulation.

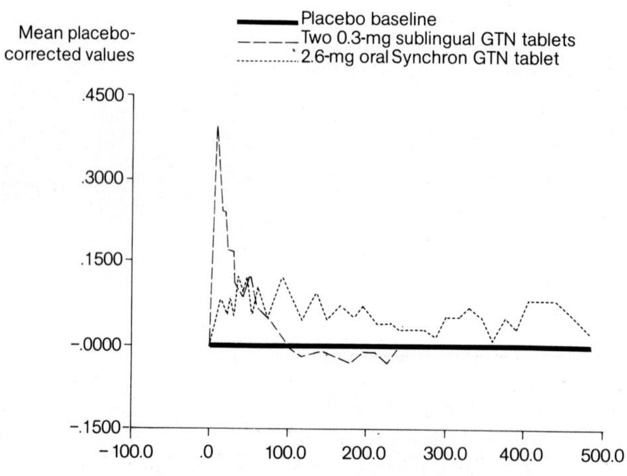

Fig. 7. Mean placebo-corrected DPG response for 0.6-mg sublingual GTN and 2.6-mg oral Synchron GTN CR tablets.

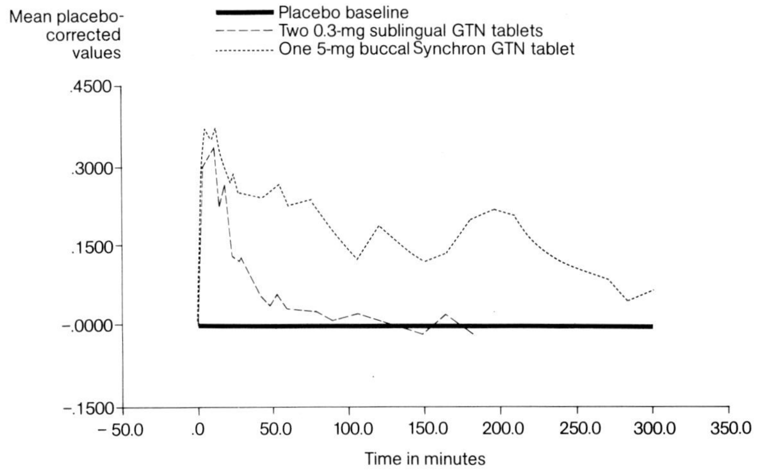

Fig. 8. Mean placebo-corrected DPG response for 0.6-mg sublingual GTN and 5-mg buccal Synchron GTN CR tablets.

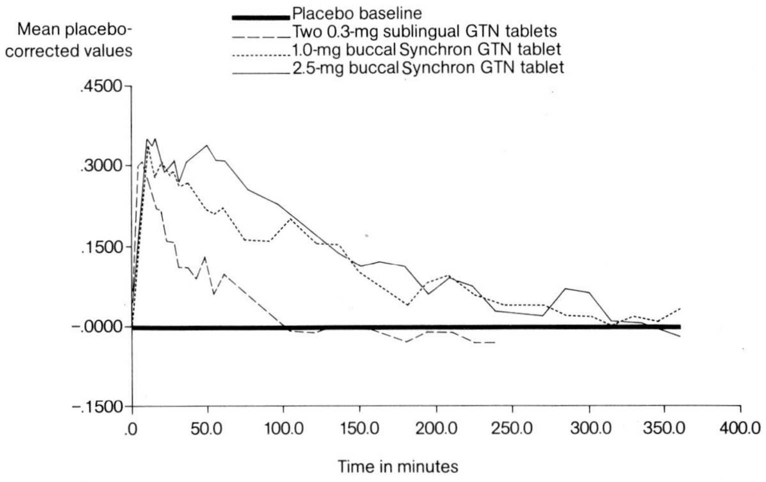

Fig. 9. Mean placebo-corrected DPG response for 0.6-mg sublingual GTN and 1.0- and 2.5-mg buccal Synchron GTN CR tablets.

Table I. Summary results of DPG studies evaluating controlled release buccal nitroglycerin dosage forms. P-C = placebo-corrected t-test duration, i.e. the number of hours the active drug is significantly different (p = 0.05) from placebo. AUC = Area under the curve

Study Number (date)	GTN Dose mg	P-C nitrostat® AUC 0–60 min	P-C peak value	P-C peak time min	t-test duration h	Number subjects	P-C AUC 0–300 min
80–27 A (4/81)	1.0	9.4	0.34	9	5	20	38.0
80–27 A (4/81)	2.5	9.4	0.35	9	5	20	46.8
77–06 (2/78)	5.0	8.9	0.37	6	4	12	53.2

Buccal Synchron GTN tablets, 1.0, 2.5, and 5.0 mg, were tested for DPG response. The first study evaluated a 5-mg dose. The DPG response was somewhat surprising in that the buccal not only produced a response which was as fast and as high as a 0.6 mg-sublingual response (fig. 8), but it also lasted for 4 h (statistically) at levels above the peak response of any of the oral dosage forms. The study was repeated using 1.0- and 2.5-mg buccal Synchron GTN doses. In this study which employed 20 (instead of 12) subjects these lower doses demonstrated statistical activity for 5 h (fig. 9).

Although the 2.5-mg dose produced an overall larger response than the 1.0-mg dose (table I), as seen by the comparison of the areas under the curve, the increase was not proportional to dose. Again, the DPG response was nearing saturation as it did in the oral study comparing the 6.5- and 10-mg doses.

References

1 Smolen, V.F.: A Study of Drug Bioavailability As Related to Physiological Response. Food and Drug Administration Contract No. 223-73-3023, 1973.

2 Federal Register, vol. 42, No. 166, August 26, 1977, pp. 43127–43131.

3 Guidelines for conducting physiologic bioavailability studies on conventional release chewable and controlled-release antianginal drug products, Division of Biopharmaceutics, Bureau of Drugs, Food and Drug Administration, August 31, 1977.

R.J. Erb, PhD, President, Pharmadynamics Research Inc.,
500 Sagamore Parkway West, West Lafayette, IN 47906 (USA)

Discussion

Chairman: *H.-L. Fung*

Fung: You have presented a very sophisticated way to measure bioavailability and I think in this case, a very pertinent way to measure one of the pharmacologic activities. One of the concerns with plethysmography has been its variability and its susceptibility to external influences. I was wondering whether you could comment on the statistical methods that you used to throw out values that are not that much higher than placebo values, given the high variability of the method?

Erb: As far as the variation goes, placebo baselines are very stable. Occasionally in the afternoon, we will find that a subject gets a little restless. We will see some oscillation. But placebo baselines normally will start at zero. We correct everything for a predrug level. They drop to a level of 0.05–0.1 units in DPG diastolic amplitude response and are very consistent for most of the day. Very rarely do we throw out data. In the studies that we have conducted since 1977, we have maybe thrown out 3 subjects we thought were artifacts; 1 we found was smoking marihuana. He had admitted to heavily smoking marihuana. He had such a tremendous response to nitrates we couldn't believe it. He had something like ten times the response of anybody else in the study. But we take it as it comes usually. We find that if you get a placebo-corrected difference of 0.1 – which is an arbitrary unit – you almost always get statistically significant results with 12–20 subjects. So it is variable, yes. But remember for you clinicians out there who are trying to correlate blood level with clinical response, you've got a problem too. I suspect that my variation is comparable to the clinical.

Wagner: I would like to know if you have correlated your bioavailability data with the nitroglycerin plasma level determinations?

Erb: I am sure that there will be a correlation...

Fung: I think there is a paper by Dr. *Imhof* in the *European Journal of Clinical Pharmacology* which shows a correlation between plasma nitroglycerin with one of the several parameters in finger plethysmography.

Schor: I think another important question is how this DPG correlates with clinical efficacy. We find the correlation to be very good in that the buccal preparation gave a very good response on a DPG which was higher than that obtained with the oral tablet, and clinically we found that the buccal tablet does produce a stronger clinical response. We get a much larger increase in exercise tolerance time with the buccal than we do with the orals although we do see significant activity with the orals. In short, the relative intensities show up very clearly in the DPG and correlate with the clinical results.

Adv. Pharmacother., vol. 1, pp. 44–48 (Karger, Basel 1982)

Nitroglycerin Blood Level after Buccal and Oral Application of Synchron Nitroglycerin

A. Windorfer

Biodesign, Institut für klinische Pharmakologie, Freiburg i.Br., FRG

The well-known effects of nitrates, particularly glyceryl trinitrate (GTN), on the vascular system (e.g. venodilatation, coronary vasodilatation, cardiac stimulation) create a specific problem in administering these drugs. On the one hand, GTN is largely and rapidly absorbed from the oral mucous membrane after sublingual application with an onset of action after 2–5 min and a maximum action after 15 min. On the other hand, 20–30 min later hardly any residual drug action is registered, a fact shown by *Abrams* [1] and *Armstrong* et al. [2]. In this short time span an acute anginal attack can be relieved but in long-term treatment significance is nil.

To cope with this problem, a number of studies on oral formulations and sustained release GTN drugs were carried out; most, however, resulting in contradictory and often negative findings and interpretations. Above all, *Needleman and Johnson* [3] postulated the first-pass effect of GTN, and due to this extensive degradation in the liver and subsequent inadequate plasma concentration, he denied these agents any clinical value.

Abrams [1] achieved significant positive results after a high dosage of oral GTN, possibly due to exhausting the hepatic metabolism, in particular, hepatic nitroreductase.

In 1977 a study with healthy volunteers was carried out comparing GTN retard tablets and GTN ointment. After the application of 2.5 mg GTN tablets an average maximum serum concentration of 0.4–0.5 ng/ml was reached after 30 min. 2 h later average serum concentrations of 0.2 ng/ml could still be detected.

We report here on a new study on the buccal application of 2.5 mg GTN tablets. In 10 patients a 2.5-mg dose was administered for 10 min and blood samples for the determination of GTN levels were taken after 4 and 10 min.

Afterwards the tablets were removed from the gum and blood samples again taken after 4 and 10 min. At the end of these 10 min a second GTN dose was administered but this time as a sublingual 0.8-mg formulation, again followed by blood sampling for GTN level determination after 4 and 10 min. Figure 1 shows the blood concentration curves:

After buccal application 7 out of 9 patients had maximum GTN concentrations varying between 0.6 and 1.5 ng/ml and 2 patients exceedingly high blood levels of 2.5 and 3.6 ng/ml.

10 min after tablet removal GTN concentrations between 0.1 and 0.5 ng/ml could clearly be identified.

After sublingual application the serum peak level was slightly higher than after buccal application followed, however, by a more rapid fall. Only in 1 patient was the blood concentration distinctly higher than the average after buccal delivery and exceedingly so after sublingual application.

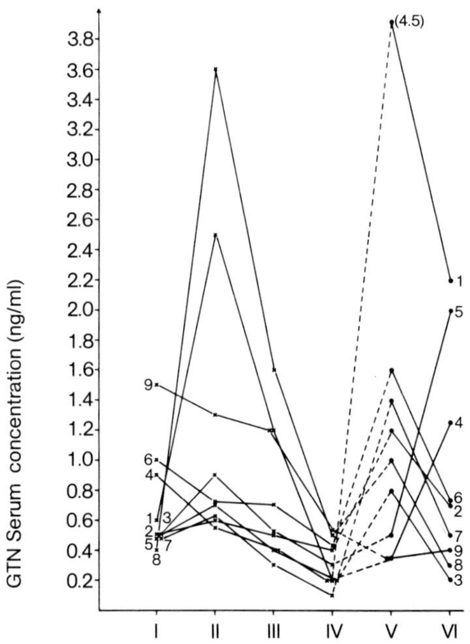

Fig. 1. Serum concentrations of GTN in adults after buccal and sublingual administration. Blood concentration curves: I = 4 min after buccal application; II = 10 min after buccal application; III = 4 min after tablet removal; IV = 10 min after tablet removal; V = 4 min after sublingual application; VI = 10 min after sublingual application.

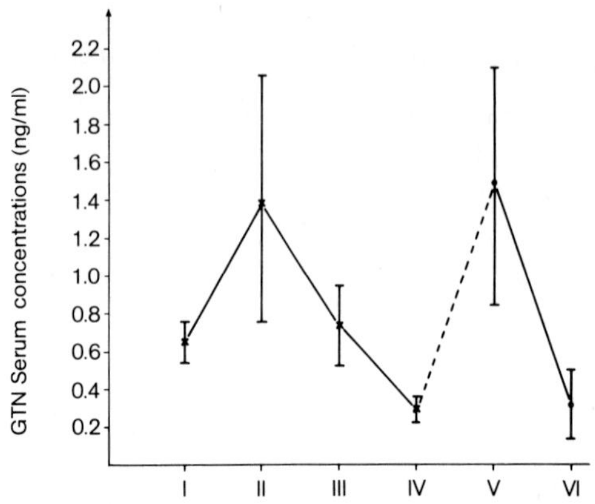

Fig. 2. Serum concentrations of GTN in adults after buccal and sublingual administration. Blood concentration curves: I = 4 min after buccal application; II = 10 min after buccal application; III = 4 min after tablet removal; IV = 10 min after tablet removal; V = 4 min after sublingual application; VI = 10 min after sublingual application.

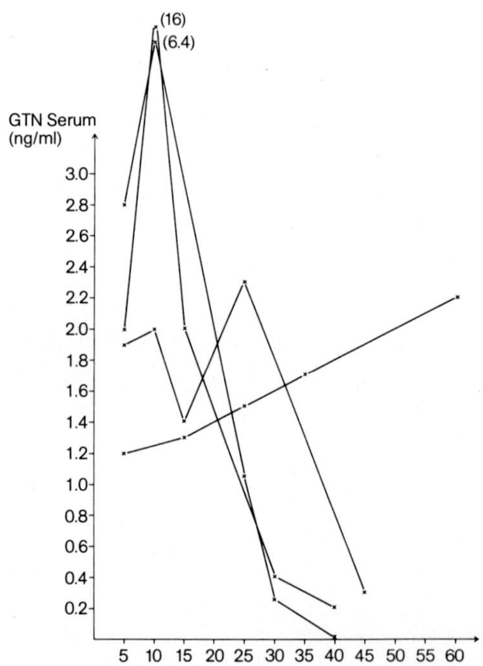

Fig. 3. GTN serum concentration of 4 patients after the administration of GTN buccal tablets. The patients kept the tablets for a different length of time between 10 and 60 min. The consumption of the tablets differed from 25% to total consumption.

The higher GTN blood concentration after sublingual application and its faster decrease in comparison with the buccal formulation indicate a slower release rate of buccal sustained release GTN (fig. 2).

Figure 3 shows the plasma concentration curves of 4 patients after buccal application of sustained release GTN for various periods of time: Subject 1 – tablet application for 30 min, complete dissolution after removal. Subject 2 – complete dissolution of tablet after 10 min. Subject 3 – 25% dissolution after 37 min. Subject 4 – 70% dissolution after 60 min.

This gives evidence of the fact that the duration of action is more prolonged after the buccal GTN application than after the sublingual one.

References

1 Abrams, J.: Usefulnes of long-acting nitrates in cardiovascular diseases (editorial). Am. J. Med. *64:* 183 (1978).

2 Armstrong, P.W.; Armstrong, J.A.; Marks, G.S.: Blood levels after sublingual nitroglycerin. Circulation *59:* 585 (1979).

3 Needleman, P.; Johnson, E.M., Jr.: Mechanism of tolerance development to organic nitrates. J. Pharmac. exp. Ther. *184:* 709 (1973).

A. Windorfer, MD, Biodesign, Institut für klinische Pharmakologie,
Carl-Mez-Strasse 81–83, D-7800 Freiburg i.Br. (FRG)

Discussion

Chairmen: *J. Abrams* and *H.J. Becker*

Lehmann: I would like to ask Dr. *Windorfer* something about the sensitivity of the concentration test.

Windorfer: Certainly, Dr. *Fung* had a higher sensitivity than we did, being able to measure concentrations down to 50 pg. Our lowest qualitative sensitivity was about 100. This is the range where we can demonstrate GTN, but we cannot differentiate between a concentration of 100 and 120 pg. Quantitative accuracy starts with us at 200 pg.

Fung: I think the assay is a difficult one and there must be all kinds of safeguards that are built into the assay if multi-center studies were conducted. We have, in collaborated studies, always asked our clinical friends to blind the samples as well as putting standards along in plasma at known concentrations so that we can correct for any changes during shipment. Transit contamination could have been a problem that Dr. *Windorfer* had with some of the samples, and I think the problem could be identified by using known concentrations in blank plasma with the same patients and processing them at the same time as collections of unknown samples. I must also support Dr. *Abrams'* point about the intersubject variability and would like to add that, in some of our data that we have just finished in determining isosorbide dinitrate absorption in angina patients, we also found a great deal of variability in the pharmacokinetics; that is in the absorption of isosorbide dinitrate amongst what were clinically a group of stable angina patients. We found that the absorption of an oral dose can range for example from about 10 to 80% of a sublingual dose. However, the intra-subject variability apparently is very much smaller. We tested the effect of a standard breakfast on absorption and found no effect of food, and we find that good absorbers of ISDN without food are good absorbers with food, and poor absorbers remain poor absorbers whether or not they have food. So the intra-subject variability appeared to be considerably smaller after oral administration than inter-subject variability. Therefore, once an optimal dosing regimen has been established, I believe for that particular individual the problem of variability may not be as much a problem.

Abrams: Dr. *Windorfer,* it appeared that 7 of the patients responded with blood levels that were quite high after the buccal preparation. Was there a relationship between the response to the buccal preparation and to the sublingual in terms of blood level responses; that is, when patients or subjects had a low level after buccal, did they also have a relatively low nitroglycerin level after sublingual or is this totally variable?

Windorfer: In 1 patient we found rather high serum concentrations after buccal application and also after sublingual application. In the second patient who also had a high concentration after buccal application we found lower serum concentration after the sublingual application. But all the other 7 patients had GTN concentrations being nearly in the same range after buccal and after sublingual application.

Abrams: Does anyone have any personal experience with the question of whether an individual subject is more or less responsive in terms of blood levels on a repetitive basis or whether this is totally random?

Fung: We have some experience. We have a study now that is ongoing where patients were given the sublingual dose three times on different days to see the reproducibility and a past study in which we had tested the pharmacokinetics of orderly administered isosorbide dinitrate over a period of several months when the patients were given doses on several occasions. As I have stated before, the intra-subject variability seems to be quite small. We don't know the reason for the differences in absorption of the buccal tablet – I have not done any buccal absorption as study in detail – but in oral absorption in animals, the results of which we have published in the *Journal of Biochemical Pharmacology,* we related that variability to the intrinsic organic nitrate reductase activity. In what is believed to be a homogenous group of animals, there is a substantial difference in the intrinsic enzyme activity in the different animals. So it is quite possible that in man also the different oral absorption may be due to the different intrinsic activity of the enzyme that denatures the drug.

Adv. Pharmacother., vol. 1, pp. 49–56 (Karger, Basel 1982)

Effects of Nitroglycerin on Vasopressin Release and the Renin-Angiotensin-Aldosterone System in Man

W. Hummerich[a], *A. Konrads*[a], *G. Wambach*[a], *K.A. Meurer*[a], *R.-R. Dries*[b], *A.-F. Langbehn*[c]

[a] Medizinische Universitäts-Poliklinik, Köln; [b] Dr. Thiemann GmbH, Lünen; [c] Rehabilitationszentrum, Bad Segeberg, FRG

Introduction

We assume that hemodynamic alterations induced by vasoactive drugs lead to responses in endogenous hormonal systems controlling blood pressure and volume homeostasis. Leaving aside catecholamines, not to be discussed here, interferences with the renin-angiotensin-aldosterone system (RAAS) and vasopressin are to be expected. The vasoactive peptide angiotensin II (A II) plays a part in acute pressure control and also stimulates aldosterone secretion. Aldosterone effects sodium and water retention and is thereby involved in long-term pressure volume control. Vasopressin has primarily been considered as the main regulator of water balance but recent findings even suggest direct vasoactive properties in man under physiological conditions.

Figure 1 illustrates the main pathways of vasodilator influence on the RAAS and vasopressin secretion. They reduce pressure in the venous, low-pressure system [9] or in arterial vessels [19] or both, thus stimulating different baroreceptors. Via vagal afferents and CNS processing efferent sympathetic pathways are stimulated that, in turn, lead to a neuromediated renin stimulation. The effector hormone A II induces aldosterone secretion. In the same way a centrally mediated stimulation of vasopressin will occur in the neurohypophysis [15]. However, vasodilators can also lead to a direct renin release via stimulation of intrarenal baroreceptors [17], either by direct action on renal vasculature or by lowering systemic blood pressure. Some vasodilators, e.g. minoxidil [20], lead to direct sodium retention by a tubular mechanism.

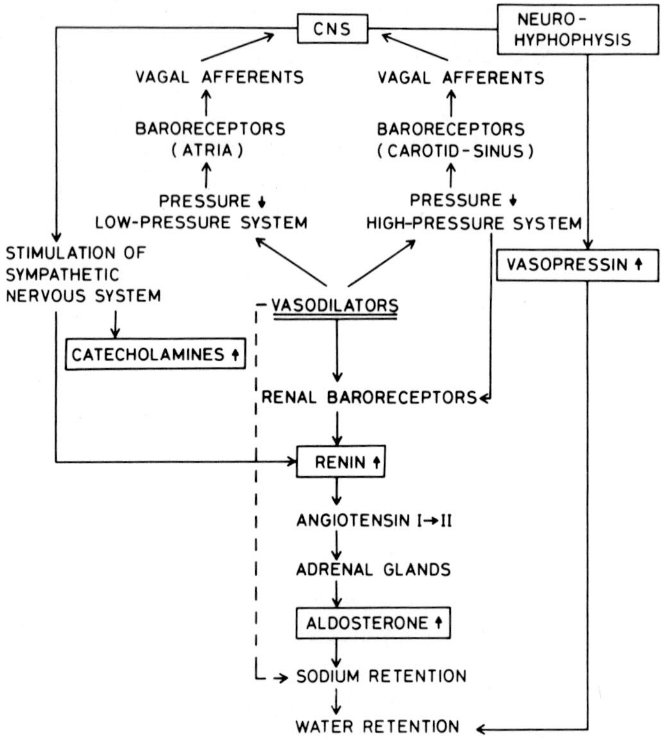

Fig. 1. Hormonal effects of vasodilator therapy.

We know from clinical experience that long-term application of some vasodilators may lead to peripheral edema by sodium and water retention. Figure 2 summarizes the most popular vasodilators. They are listed according to their action on the venous (preload) or arterial system (afterload). Sodium- and water-retaining properties have been found after minoxidil, hydralazine, diazoxide and prazosine. These effects are generally not present after nitroglycerin administration. All substances listed in figure 2 are known renin stimulators at least in acute experiments [6]. There are only a few studies on aldosterone secretion during vasodilator therapy and the results obtained are controversial [14]. No data on the RAAS or vasopressin secretion after acute or chronic treatment with nitrates in man are available.

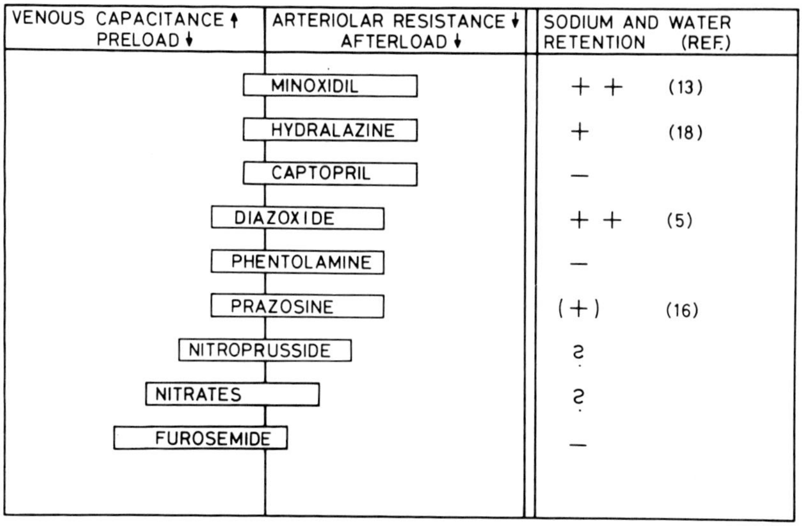

Fig. 2. Hemodynamic effects of vasodilators.

Methods

Short-Term Studies. Determinations of plasma renin concentration (PRC) and vasopressin in plasma were made 3 and 30 min after buccal application of 1–5 mg (mean 2.5 mg) of buccal Synchron nitroglycerin in patients with coronary heart disease. The results were correlated to mean pulmonary pressure (PAP) and arterial blood pressure (indirect measurement). A previous study had shown that exercise stress tests started 3 min after buccal nitroglycerin had no effect on PRC or vasopressin secretion. Plasma samples were taken from the studies of Dr. *Langbehn.* The design of his study is explained in his contribution.

Long-Term Studies. The effect of chronic nitroglycerin application on PRC and aldosterone secretion has been studied in 20 patients with coronary heart disease during long-term treatment with 5.2–20 mg (mean 12.5 mg) of a new oral Synchron nitroglycerin formulation. Plasma samples were taken after 3 and 8 weeks of treatment during the late morning hours under outpatient conditions. 24-hour urine collection for the determination of aldosterone excretion was carried out the day before.

The determination of PRC [3], vasopressin [4] and aldosterone [2] followed the established routine RIA techniques described elsewhere.

Results

Short-Term Studies. The acute effect of nitroglycerin on PRC is shown in figure 3. Patients were subdivided into 2 groups according to their response in PAP: The first group (triangles) had a decrease in PAP of more than 2 mm

3 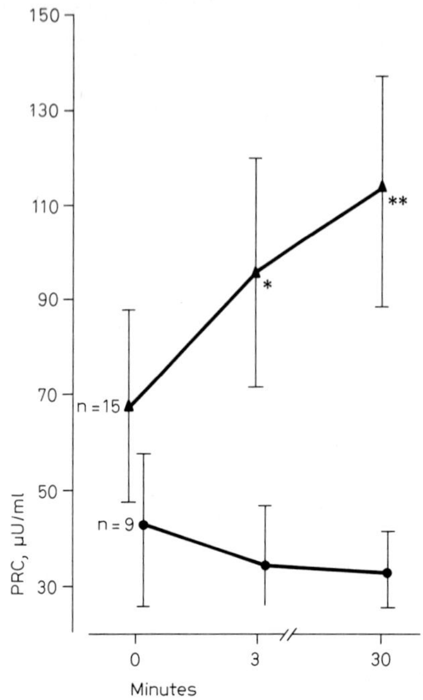

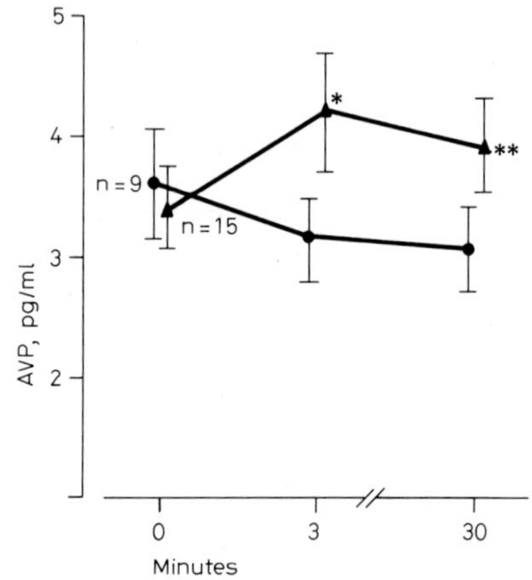 4

Fig. 3. Influence of nitroglycerin on PRC. Data are given as mean ± SEM. For evaluation of significance standard t-test procedures for paired data were used. *$p < 0.1$; **$p < 0.05$.

Fig. 4. Effects of nitroglycerin on vasopressin (AVP) release (see also fig. 3).

Hg at any time between 0 and 30 min. In the second group (closed circles) the PAP did not decrease or was less than 2 mm Hg. We observed that a significant PRC increase followed only in patients with a decrease in PAP. Figure 4 shows the corresponding results for vasopressin in the same two groups of patients. Again a significant increase in AVP was only observed in patients with a fall in PAP. The increase in PRC and AVP was not correlated to the magnitude of pressure fall and was not different in groups of patients under different dosages of nitroglycerin and thus followed an all-or-none characteristic. Linear regression analysis showed a high correlation between PRC and vasopressin increase at 30 min (linear coefficient of correlation $r = 0.8$, $p < 0.05$). As far as arterial pressure changes were concerned no differences in PRC and vasopressin could be detected in patients with or without a fall in blood pressure.

5
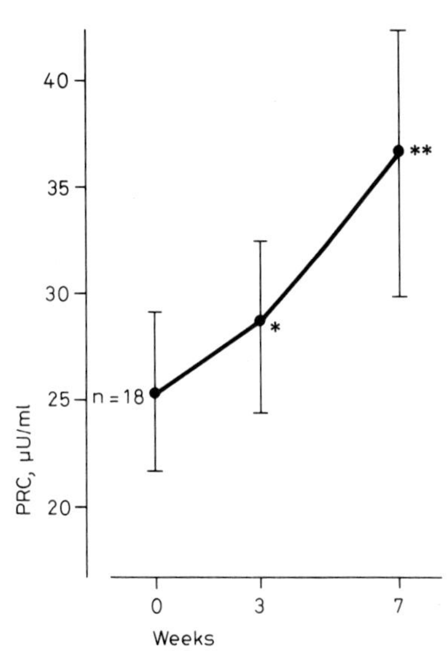

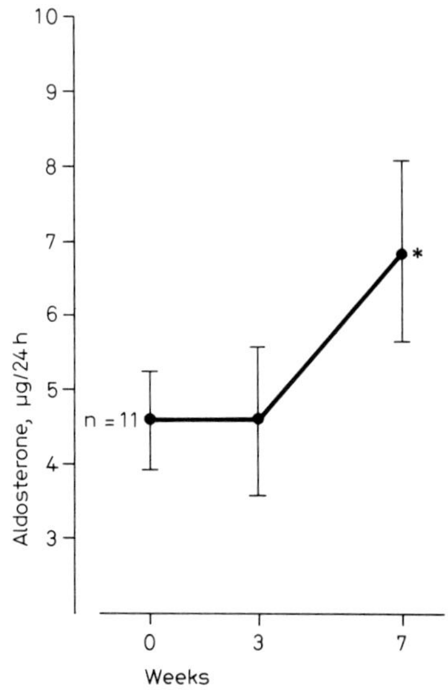

6

Fig. 5. Effects of long-term nitroglycerin treatment on PRC (see also fig. 3).

Fig. 6. Effects of long-term nitroglycerin treatment on aldosterone excretion in 24-hour urine (see also fig. 3).

Long-Term Studies. The effect of long-term nitroglycerin treatment on PRC is shown in figure 5. A significant increase was observed after 7 weeks. However, PRC peak values remained below the pathological range. Similar values could be observed after orthostasis in man. The results of aldosterone secretion are given in figure 6. Again an increase in aldosterone secretion occurs, but the difference to baseline values is only of low significance. The values are again in the normal range if correlated to sodium excretion during the urine-collection period.

Discussion

The results show that nitroglycerin induces an acute stimulation of PRC and vasopressin in plasma. This finding could have been expected as a consequence of the known nitroglycerin action on low- and high-pressure systems. Similarly, tilting maneuvers led to a stimulation of these hormones, inducing a fall in the low-pressure system by peripheral blood pooling or by decreasing cardiac output [16]. So far, there has not been any final evidence as to whether low- or high-pressure receptors dominate in this respect [19]. Our results suggest that receptors in the cardiopulmonary region might be of greater importance because no correlation to arterial blood pressure could be established.

While these problems of acute vasopressin and renin control are more theoretical in their interest value, the influence of nitroglycerin on renin and aldosterone secretion during long-term treatment is of greater practical value. A secondary hyperaldosteronism of clinical relevance can only be expected if there is sustained A II-induced stimulation of aldosterone leading to elevated hormone levels for a prolonged period of time. Such clinical situations are renal artery stenosis, abuse of laxatives or diuretics. Our results show that long-term treatment with nitroglycerin stimulates renin as well as aldosterone secretion, but the increase is small and pathologically elevated levels are not observed. Thus, a relevant secondary hyperaldosteronism can be excluded in the patients studied. To our knowledge no renin and aldosterone measurements have yet been performed under long-term therapy with nitrates in man. *Kraupp* et al. [7] investigated whether application of nitrates in dogs for 5 days led to renin stimulation and they only found a minor increase in renin secretion. In contrast to other vasoactive agents, a sodium-retaining effect or development of edema is generally not observed under nitroglycerin in man. This may be the reason why detailed examination of sodium and water balance during application of these drugs in man has not been performed. However, the situation may be different in patients with heart failure. Some observations in patients with congestive heart failure, elevated pulmonary pressures and oliguria have shown that application of isosorbide dinitrate (ISDN) induced diuresis and natriuresis [10]. It was assumed that nitrates improved renal blood flow in these cases. It is well-known from animal experiments that acute application of nitroglycerin induces a local increase in renal blood flow [8, 12]. By contrast, a subgroup of patients with severe cardiac failure, low cardiac output, and low arterial blood pressure has been described as developing ascites after ISDN, resistant to furosemide but with good response to the aldosterone antagonist spironolactone [10]. It was argued that in these cases a fall in cardiac output reduced the renal perfusion pressure leading to renin and aldosterone stimulation via renal baroreceptors. It is known that in severe congestive heart failure with edema, renal blood flow is reduced [11] and may be further diminished when nitrates lead to an additional fall in systemic blood pressure. If these hemodynamic situations are excluded it may be assumed that under normal conditions a significant renin release and secondary hyperaldosteronism do not occur because local vasodilating actions of nitrates tend to improve renal blood flow and thus suppress renin secretion or at least compensate for concomitant renin-releasing mechanisms.

References

1 Brennan, L.A.; Malvin, R.L.; Jochim, K.F.; Roberts, D.E.: Influence of right and left atrial receptors on plasma concentrations of ADH and renin. Am. J. Physiol. *221:* 273–278 (1971).

2 Helber, A.; Kaufmann, W.: Radioimmunologische Methode zur Aldosteronbestimmung im Urin. Klin. Wschr. *51:* 1164–1169 (1973).

3 Hummerich, W.; Krause, D.K.: Improvement of renin determination in human plasma using a commonly available renin standard in a radioimmunological method. Klin. Wschr. *53:* 559–571 (1975).

4 Hummerich, W.; Konrads, A.; Sofroniew, M.: Radioimmunoassay of argenin vasopressin in human plasma. Methodological aspects and clinical application (submitted for publication).

5 Hutcheon, D.E.; Barthalmus, K.S.: Antihypertensive action of diazoxide. Br. med. J. *ii:* 159–161 (1962).

6 Johnston, C.I.: Effect of antihypertensive drugs on the renin-angiotensin system. Drugs *12:* 274–291 (1976).

7 Kraupp, O.; Benke, T.; Placheta, P.; Stapek, B.; Raberger, G.: Die Wirkung einer einmaligen sowie chronischen Verabreichung von Isoket auf die Plasma-Renin-Aktivität von Hunden; in Rudolph, Schrey, Nitrate II, 2. Nitrat Symp., Berlin, pp. 17–21 (Urban & Schwarzenberg, München 1980).

8 Maldinzak, G.S.; Schmidt, H.; McCurdy, J.: Vasodilator response in the ischemic kidney. Circulation *40:* suppl. 3, p. 138 (1969).

9 Mancia, G.; Romero, J.C.; Sheperd, J.T.: Continuous inhibition of renin release in dogs by vagally innervated receptors in the cardiopulmonary region. Circulation Res. *36:* 529–535 (1975).

10 Mantle, J.A.; Russel, R.O.; Rogers, W.J.; Rackley, C.E.: Renal effects of ISDN in congestive heart failure complicating myocardial infarction; in Rudolph, Schrey, Nitrate II, 2. Nitrat Symp., Berlin, pp. 17–21 (Urban & Schwarzenberg, München 1980).

11 Merril, A.J.: Edema and decreased renal blood flow in patients with chronic congestive heart failure. J. clin. Invest. *25:* 389–400 (1946).

12 Oguro, K.; Hashinoto, K.: Quantitative and comparative studies of pharmalogical features in the coronary, femoral and renal circulations with different coronary vasodilators. Jap. J. Pharmacol. *24:* 227–233 (1974).

13 Pettinger, W.A.: Minoxidil and the treatment of severe hypertension. New Engl. J. Med. *303:* 922–926 (1980).

14 Pratt, H.J.; Yayer, C.J.; Grim, C.E.; Parkinson, C.A.: Increased aldosterone metabolic clearance in hypertensive patients treated with minoxidil. J. cardiovasc. Pharmacol. *2:* suppl. 2, p. 236 (1980).

15 Rocha e Silva, M.; Celso de Lima, W.; Castro de Souza, E.M.: Vasopressin secretion in response to hemorrhage. Pflügers Arch. *376:* 185–190 (1978).

16 Thulin, T.; Saetre, H.; Vikesdahl, O.; Warmenius, S.; Persson, G.: Multicenter study of the antihypertensive effect of prazosine on mild and moderate hypertension, pp. 126–137 (Excerpta Medica, Amsterdam 1974).
17 Vander, A.J.; Carlson, J.: Mechanism of the effects of furosemide on renin secretion in anesthetized dogs. Circulation Res. *24:* 145–152 (1969).
18 Zacest, R.; Gilmous, E.; Koch-Weser, J.: Treatment of essential hypertension with combined vasodilation and beta-adrenergic blockade. New Engl. J. Med. *286:* 617–620 (1972).
19 Zanchetti, A.; Stella, A.; Dampney, R.: Central and reflex control of renin release. Prog. Brain Res. *47:* 397–409 (1977).
20 Zins, G.R.: Alterations in renal function during vasodilator therapy; in Laurend, Wesson, Recent advances in renal physiology and pharmacology (Medical & Technical Publishing, Lancaster 1974).

W. Hummerich, MD, Medizinische Universitäts-Poliklinik, Josef-Stelzmann-Strasse 9, D-5000 Köln 41 (FRG)

Discussion

Chairmen: *U. Gleichmann* and *N. Reichek*

Reichek: Dr. *Hummerich,* there has been at least one report in the American literature of systematic differences in the hemodynamic response to nitrates in heart failure patients who are volume-overloaded as contrasted to those who are not volume-overloaded and do not have peripheral edema at the time the agent is administered. Can you relate that to the effects that you've demonstrated on the renin-angiotensin system?

Hummerich: No. The only observation in that respect I know about was made by *Mantle* et al. [10]. It must be stressed that in these cases only ascites and not peripheral edema developed; so there must have been some additional factors. May I ask the audience whether anybody has observed sodium or water retention under nitrates in man?

Bussmann: We used 120 mg of isosorbid dinitrate per day in patients with chronic heart failure, high filling pressure and low cardiac output. We didn't ever oberserve any water retention or increase in peripheral edema. This was seen following prazosine and other substances which act more on the arterial side. You mentioned that the stimulation of renin and angiotensin secretion is not as extensive to result in pathological changes?

Hummerich: That's right. But we didn't study patients with congestive heart failure. The situation may really be different in a subgroup of patients with congestive heart failure, which might have a preexisting stimulation of the renin-angiotensin system. If there are additional influences, for example nitroglycerin or similar drugs, that might further stimulate the renin-angiotensin system it might be that in these cases edema develops.

Adv. Pharmacother., vol. 1, pp. 57–63 (Karger, Basel 1982)

Hemodynamics and Lung Function in Patients with Chronic Obstructive Lung Disease following Administration of Nitroglycerin and Aminophylline

B. Niehues, R. Thoma

Universität Köln, Medizinische Klinik III und I (Direktoren: Prof. Dr. *H.H. Hilger*, Prof. Dr. *R. Gross*), Köln, FRG

Chronic obstructive lung disease (COLD) usually results in progressive increase of pressure in the pulmonary artery, leading to right heart failure in the terminal course of the disease. Additionally to the von Euler-Liljestrand mechanism vascular resistance is enhanced by the increased intrathoracic pressure induced by mechanical impairment of the ventilation especially during the exspiratory phase. The aim of this study was to acquire some information concerning the extent and the means by which nitroglycerin (GTN) may influence pulmonary hemodynamics and ventilation and to compare these results with the effects of aminophylline (APH).

Patients, Methods and Results

In a first series 12 patients with an average age of 60 years were investigated. Broncholytic therapy was discontinued the evening prior to the investigation. Pulmonary function testing was performed 24 h before and after the hemodynamic studies. The following parameters were obtained both at rest and during exercise in the supine position (0.5 W/kg BW) before and after administration of GTN (0.8 mg sublingually): heart rate, blood pressure, phasic and mean pulmonary artery pressure (floating catheter), cardiac output (Fick principle); respiratory oscillations were monitored over three respiratory cycles. At rest and after administration of 0.8 mg GTN the following parameters were measured in the pulmonary function laboratory by whole body plethysmography: total lung capacity (TLC), vital capacity (VC), functional residual capacity (FRC), respiratory volume (RV), forced exspi-

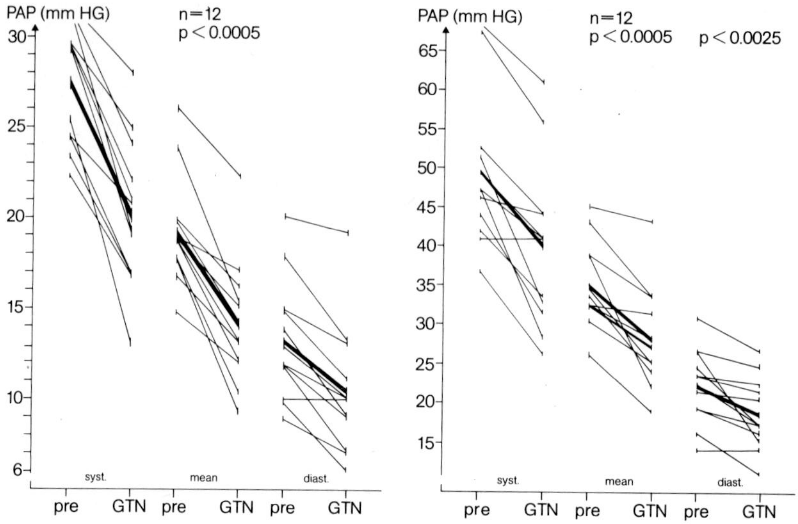

Fig. 1. Phasic and mean pulmonary artery pressure (PAP) at rest (left) and during exercise (right) before and after administration of nitroglycerin (GTN).

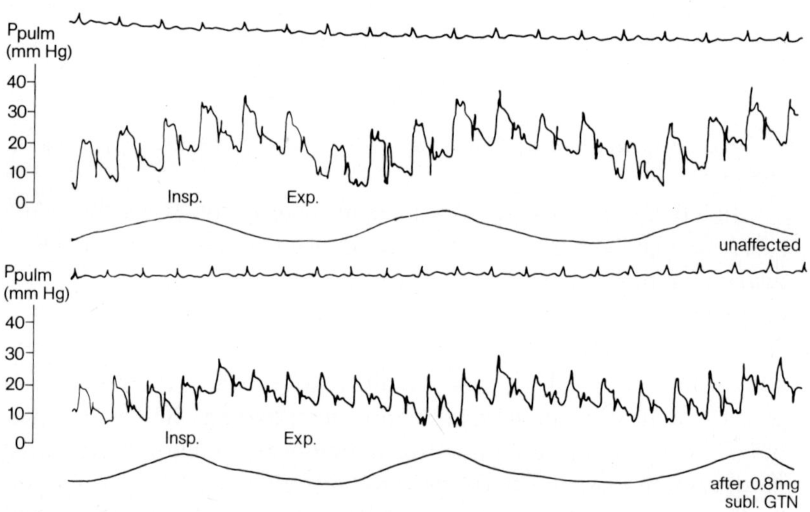

Fig. 2. Respiratory-dependent oscillations of the PAP before (upper chanel) and after administration of GTN.

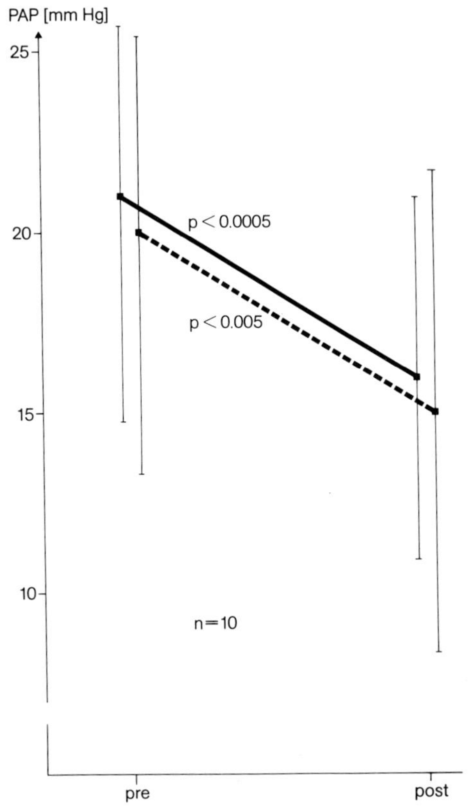

Fig. 3. Changes of PAP before and after application of GTN (——) and APH (– – –).

ratory volume in the first second (FEV_1), airway resistance, and partial pressures of O_2 and CO_2.

After GTN cardiac output decreased from 5.1 to 4.2 l/min, corresponding to a fall of 16%, the mean pulmonary artery pressure decreased from 20 to 14 mm Hg. During ergometric exercise prior to GTN, mean pulmonary arterial pressure increased to 34 mm Hg, following GTN there was an increase to only 28 mm Hg (fig. 1). The respiratory-dependent oscillations of the pulmonary artery pressure, normally not exceeding 5 mm Hg, extended to 13 mm Hg both during systole and diastole. The enhanced airway obstruction during the exspiratory phase increases the intrathoracic pressure resulting in a more pronounced respiratory pressure oscillation. These oscillations were significantly reduced after administration of GTN (fig. 2). With respect

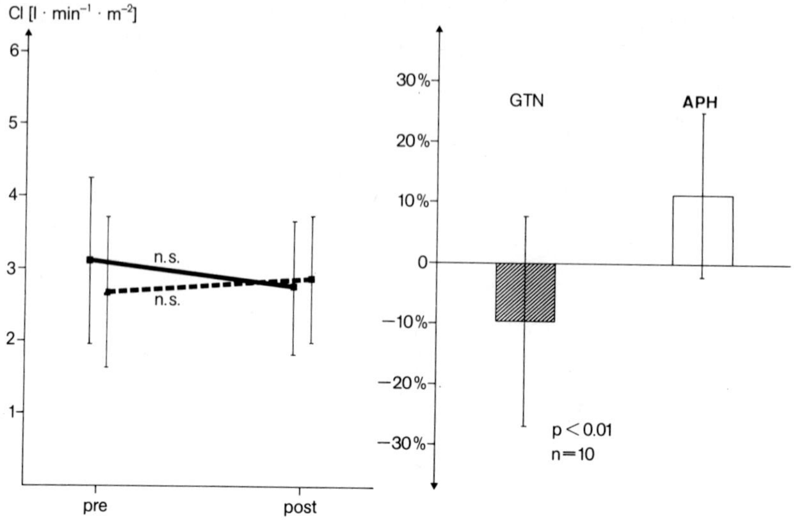

Fig. 4. Changes of cardiac index (CI) before and after application of GTN (——) and APH (– – –) and percentual changes after administration of the drugs.

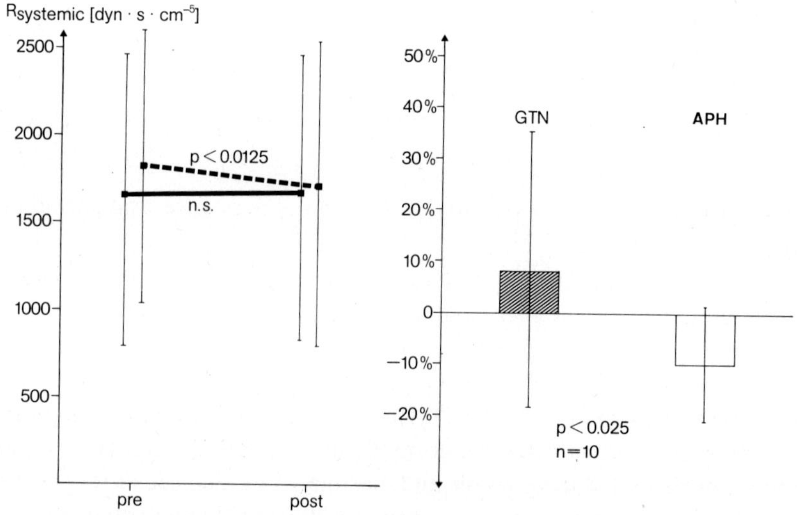

Fig. 5. Changes of systemic resistance after application of GTN (——) and APH (– – –) and percentual changes after administration of the drugs.

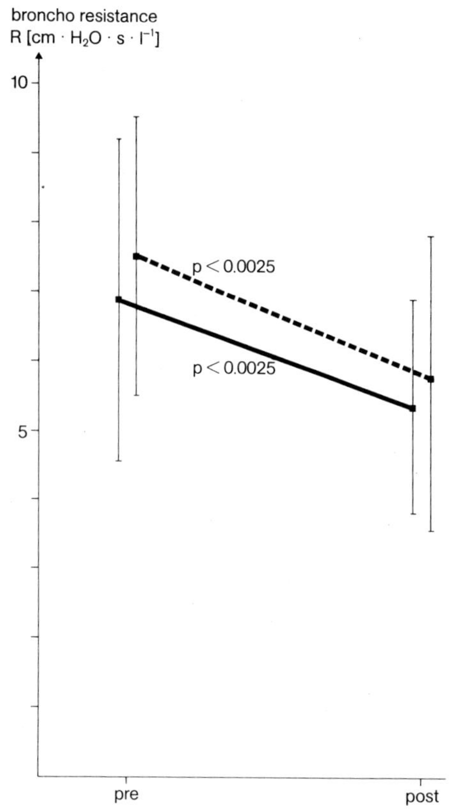

Fig. 6. Bronchoresistance after application of GTN (——) and APH (– – –).

to the ventilatory parameters airway resistance has diminished considerably from 5.7 to 4.1 cm $H_2O/l/s$, corresponding to an increased FEV_1. Arterial p_{O_2} and p_{CO_2} were not altered by GTN.

In a second series we examined 10 patients with an average age of 62 years in order to demonstrate the simultaneous change in lung function and hemodynamics following an oral application of 0.8 mg GTN and to compare these results with the effect of a steady-state infusion of APH, showing an equipotent reduction of the mean pulmonary artery pressure (PAP). The hemodynamic measurements were performed in the above-mentioned manner. The airway resistance was measured with SIREGNOST (Siemens) simultaneously several times before and 5 min after application of GTN. After a recovery time of 45 min we continued the examination by giving an infusion of APH in a dose of 480 mg over 20 min. A steady state was obtained with further 240 mg APH over 100 min. The simultaneous measurements of hemodynamic and airway resistance was performed 60 min following the start of APH.

Following GTN there was a decrease of PAP from 22 to 16 mm Hg. During the infusion of APH we observed a nearly identical change in the PAP from 20 to 15 mm Hg (fig. 3). Looking at the cardiac index there was a moderate decrease from 3.1 to 2.7 $l/min/m^2$ following GTN and a slight increase from 2.6 to 2.8 $l/min/m^2$ following APH. A significant difference between the percentage changes could be found, showing a decrease of 9% after GTN and an increase of 11% following APH (fig. 4). Regarding the systemic resistance GTN did not cause a change, whereas during the infusion of APH we observed a diminution from 1,823 to 1,679 $dyn \times s \times cm^{-5}$. There was a significant difference between the percentage changes of the two drugs (fig. 5). Bronchoresistance measured simultaneously with the hemodynamics revealed an equal decrease from 7 to 5.4 units following GTN and from 7.5 to 5.7 units following APH (fig. 6).

Discussion

The influence of nitrates on pulmonary ventilation and gas exchange has only been evaluated in the last few years. In 10 patients with cor pulmonale *Konietzko* et al. [3] reported a 4-mm Hg decrease of the arterial p_{O_2} and an increased alveoloarterial difference of p_{O_2} after administration of ISDN. These results were confirmed by *Goeckenjan and Barthels* [1] and *Kochukoshy* et al. [2]. Their results were explained by pulmonary vasodilatation counteracting the von Euler-Liljestrand mechanism. However, we were not able to measure any GTN-induced alteration of the arterial p_{O_2} as a mean. The improvement of the pulmonary ventilation is documented by the considerable decrease of the respiratory pressure oscillations in the pulmonary artery as well as by the significant reduction of airway resistance. The intrathoracic pressure is lowered by reduction of airway resistance and the pulmonary vascular resistance is diminished, thus resulting in a decrease of PAP.

GTN acts predominantly on the postcapillary vessels, leading to a venous pooling with decrease of the cardiac output. GTN produces venodilatation, and the morphology of the pulmonary vascular bed equals the venous system.

In contrast APH acts on the precapillary vessels with a decrease of systemic resistance and an increase of cardiac output, but equal responses to PAP and airway resistance. The decrease of airway resistance by both GTN and APH must be explained by direct action on the bronchi.

References

1 Goeckenjan, G.; Barthels, F.: Pulmonaler Gasaustausch unter einer Behandlung mit Nitroglyzerin. Verh. dt. Ges. Lungen-Atemwegsforsch. *6:* 187 (1976).

2 Kochukoshy, K.N.; Chick, T.W.; Jenne, J.W.: The effect of nitroglycerin on gas exchange in chronic obstructive pulmonary disease. Am. Rev. resp. Dis. *11:* 177 (1975).

3 Konietzko, N.; Schlehe, H.; Härlich, B.; Matthys, H.: Effect of isosorbide dinitrate on hemodynamics and respiration of patients with coronary artery disease and of patients with chronic cor pulmonale. Respiration *32:* 368 (1975).

B. Niehues, MD, Medizinische Klinik III und I, Josef-Stelzmann-Strasse, D-5000 Köln 41 (FRG)

Adv. Pharmacother., vol. 1, pp. 64–72 (Karger, Basel 1982)

Acute Hemodynamic and Pharmacokinetic Effects of Buccal Nitroglycerin

Wulf-Dirk Bussmann, Walter Kromm, Nikolaus Reifart, Ho-Leung Fung

Center of Internal Medicine, Department of Cardiology, University Clinic of the Johann Wolfgang Goethe University, Frankfurt am Main, FRG; Department of Pharmaceutics, State University of New York at Buffalo, Buffalo, N.Y., USA

We investigated 19 patients with coronary heart disease during diagnostic heart catherization.

In the first study protocol, 11 patients received 2.5 mg of buccal Synchron nitroglycerin before the procedure began and any contrast material had been injected. The patients were told to put the tablet in the buccal region and not to move. After 10 min, the tablet was removed and a washout period of 10 min allowed. Then 0.8 mg of nitroglycerin were administered sublingually and measurements were repeated for another 10 min. Heart rate, aortic pressure and left ventricular systolic and enddiastolic pressure were measured every 2 min. Blood samples for determination of plasma nitroglycerin concentration were taken during the 4th and 10th minute of each phase. The samples were kept in icewater, plasma was separated within 30 min using a refrigerated centrifuge and were rapidly frozen. Care was taken to analyze samples as soon as possible, that is within 2–3 weeks. Samples were analyzed parallel in Dr. *Fung's* laboratory, Buffalo, N.Y. (USA) and by the Biodesign Institute, Freiburg (FRG). No difference exists between the two.

In the second protocol 12 patients had a coronary angiography before and after 1.0–2.5 mg of buccal nitroglycerin. Coronary diameters were measured in the left and right coronary artery at the same anatomical location by unbiased observer. The film was projected on a screen at a distance of 100 cm. In 3 of these patients plasma concentrations were measured over a period of 60 min.

First we looked at the dissolution rate of the buccal tablet in relation to nitroglycerin plasma levels. After 10 min 2 patients dissolved their tablets completely despite the instructions not to move with the tablet inside the mouth. In the medium group 40% of the tablet was gone and in the slow dissolution group about 20%. The loss of tablet mass was judged arbitrarily by comparison with an original tablet (fig. 1).

The highest blood levels were obtained in those patients in whom the tablet was dissolved within 10 min. The plasma concentration was 14 ng/ml. In the two other groups more favorable blood levels were obtained. This has the clinical implication that the buccal tablet should not be moved too much in the mouth to avoid peak plasma concentration and possible side effects. Dissolution rate is more rapid in the presence of more movement and salivation.

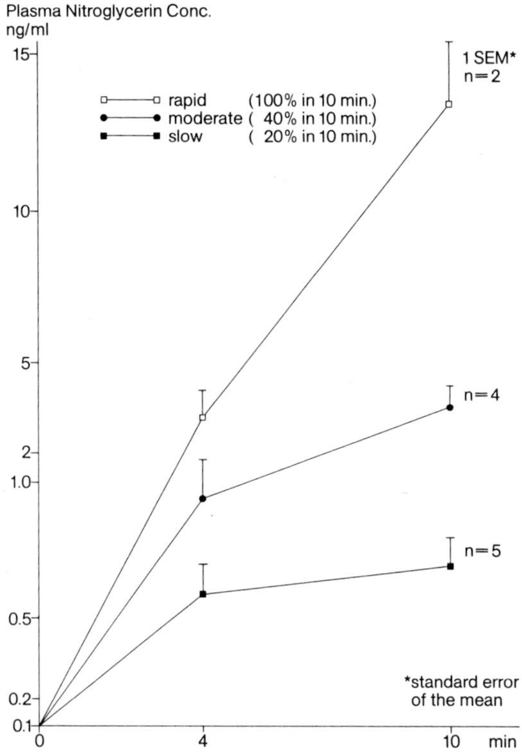

Fig. 1. 2 patients dissolved their tablets within 10 min. Plasma concentration reached 14 ng/ml. In the medium group 40% of the tablet was dissolved and much lower plasma levels were observed. In the third group 20% of the tablets were dissolved. Here the lowest plasma nitroglycerin concentrations were found.

2
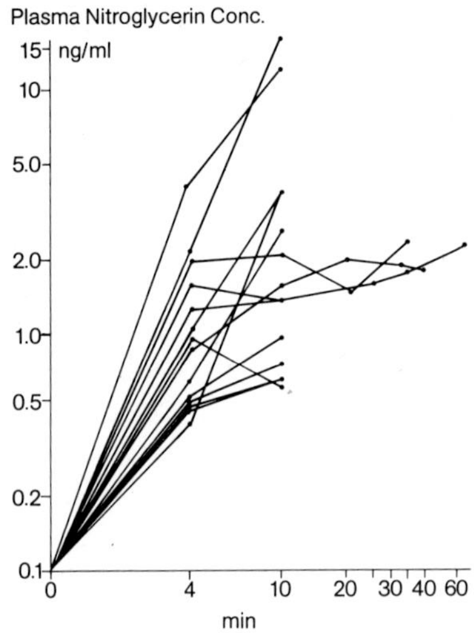

3
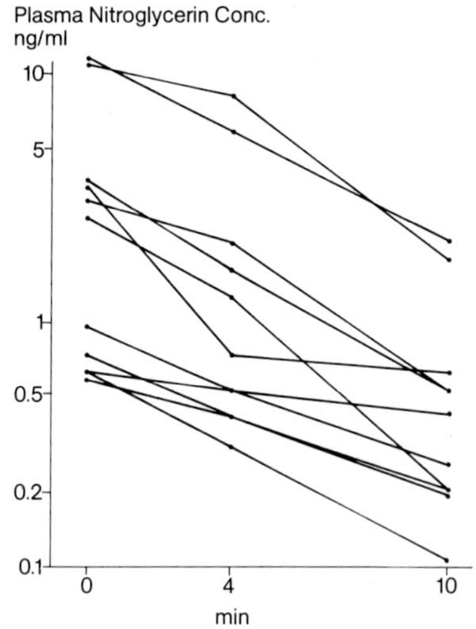

Fig. 2. Plasma nitroglycerin concentration is plotted versus time, both in logarithmic scales. A plateau is reached after 10 min. It seems to be stable thereafter for up to 60 min, at least in the 3 cases shown.

Fig. 3. After removal of the buccal tablet a rapid drop of plasma nitroglycerin concentration was observed. Elimination half-time was 5–6 min.

Figure 2 shows again plasma nitroglycerin concentration plotted versus time following 2.5 mg of buccal nitroglycerin in logarithmic scales. A plateau is reached after 10 min and seems to be stable thereafter, as evident from 3 cases, who were observed for 60 min.

It is well known that nitroglycerin is rapidly eliminated from the plasma (fig. 3). We calculated an elimination half-time of about 5–6 min. In 10 min 75% is eliminated [1–3].

The acute hemodynamic effects of 2.5 mg of buccal nitroglycerin are shown in figure 4. Heart rate increased slightly during the 10-min observation period. Left ventricular enddiastolic pressure decreased significantly with the absolute decrease most pronounced in those patients with filling pressure above 20 mm Hg. In those left ventricular filling pressure decreased from 25 to 14 mm Hg. Arterial pressure dropped by 16 mm Hg systolic and only 3 mm Hg diastolic. In patients with initially high blood pressure the decrease was more pronounced.

The dose-effect relationship can be seen from figure 5. 1.0 mg was compared with 2.5 mg of buccal nitroglycerin. 2.5 mg had a greater effect than

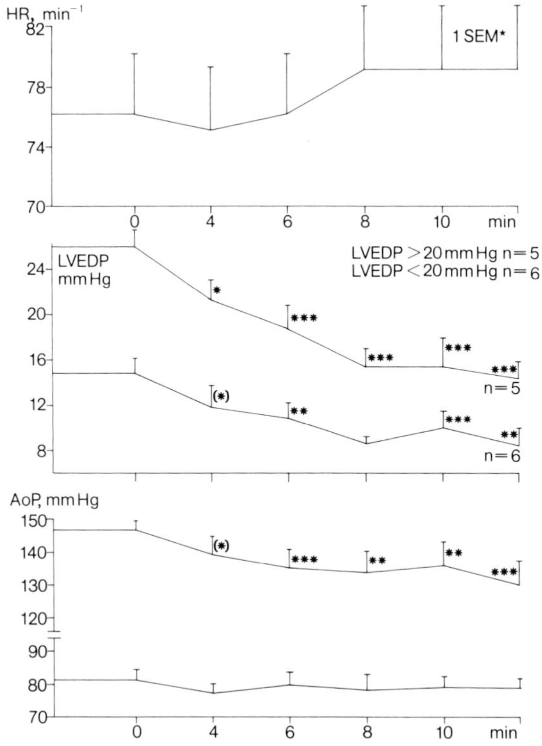

Fig. 4. 2.5 mg of buccal nitroglycerin produced a slight but not significant increase in heart rate. Left ventricular enddiastolic pressure decreased significantly both in patients with and without left ventricular failure (below and above 20 mm Hg). Systolic arterial pressure decreased by 16 mm Hg, diastolic arterial pressure by 3 mm Hg. $^{(*)}p < 0.1$; $^{*}p < 0.05$; $^{**}p < 0.025$; $^{***}p < 0.005$.

1.0 mg. This was evaluated in patients with a left ventricular filling pressure above 20 mm Hg.

Coronary diameter, as measured following protocol 2, increased by a mean of 17% in the left and 7% in the right coronary artery (fig. 6). These values are comparable to the effect of sublingual nitroglycerin.

The comparison of buccal to sublingual nitroglycerin is shown in figure 7. The buccal tablet was left in the patient's mouth for 10 min, the washout period lasted 10 min and then sublingual nitroglycerin was investigated for another 10 min. Plasma concentration as shown in the upper panel illustrates this protocol nicely: There is an increase in the concentration within the first 10 min and a fall in the washout phase. Following administration of sublin-

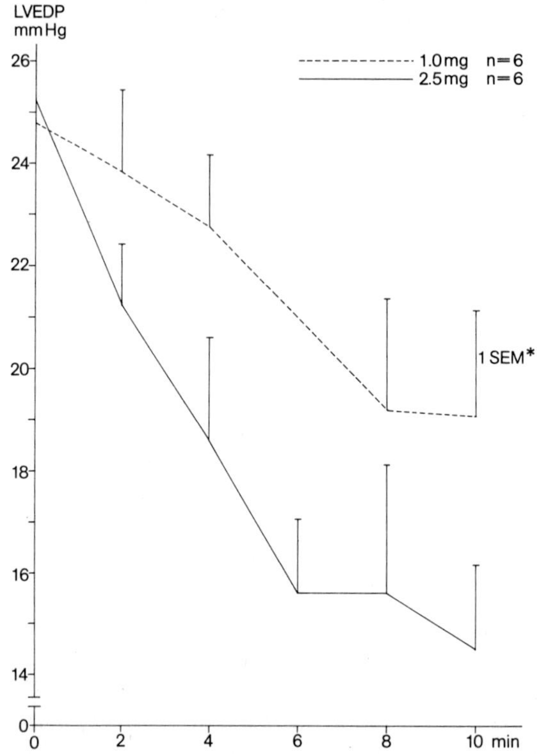

Fig. 5. Effect of 1.0 and 2.5 mg of buccal nitroglycerin on left ventricular enddiastolic pressure. The effect was more pronounced in patients receiving 2.5 mg. This was evaluated in patients with left ventricular filling pressure above 20 mm Hg.

gual nitroglycerin, another increase was observed. The hemodynamic response can clearly be seen following the first nitroglycerin application: Left ventricular enddiastolic pressure decreased significantly and there was a mild decrease of systolic and diastolic aortic pressure. During the washout period, however, the control values were not reached. Despite the renewed increase in nitroglycerin plasma concentration, the hemodynamic response to sublingual nitroglycerin was minimal. This, however, has mainly to do with the briefness of the washout period.

From the plasma concentration data another interesting calculation can be made. Excluding the 2 patients with the rapid dissolution rate of the tablet, a plasma concentration of 1.4 ng/ml is reached when about 30% of buccal tablet is dissolved. This is related to a dose of 0.75 mg of buccal nitroglycerin.

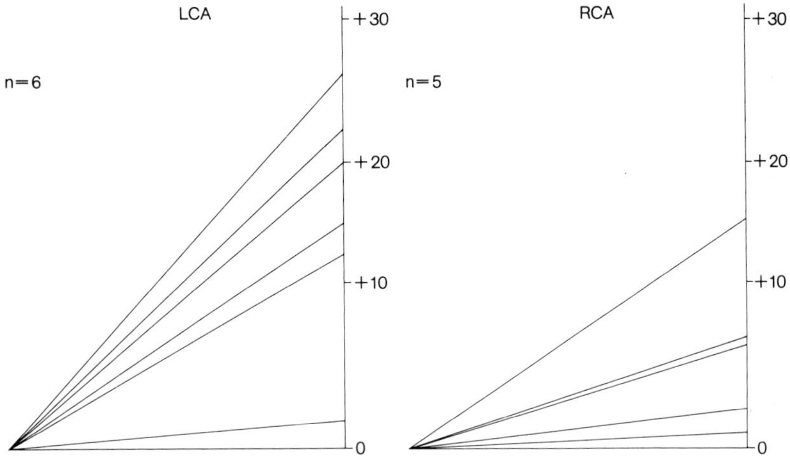

Fig. 6. Coronary diameter was measured before and after 2.5 mg of buccal nitroglycerin. Both in the left (LCA) and the right coronary artery (RCA) coronary diameter increased. Measurements were taken from the same location and same projection of the large epicardial arteries.

Following 0.8 mg of sublingual nitroglycerin nearly the same plasma level of 1.3 ng/ml is reached. Thus, the same absolute amount of nitroglycerin, whether administered buccally or sublingually, results nearly in the same plasma concentration.

In conclusion, effective plasma levels are reached at least within 4 min following buccal nitroglycerin. Hemodynamic effects in terms of a reduction in left ventricular filling pressure and decrease in systolic arterial pressure are evident within 2 min. After 10 min a plateau in the plasma concentration is reached. Only in those patients who moved the buccal tablet in their mouth were extremely high levels reached. Increasing the dose from 1 to 2.5 mg of nitroglycerin led to a more pronounced decrease in left ventricular enddiastolic pressure. Dilatation of the epicardial coronary arteries, ranging from 7 to 17%, could also be shown clearly after buccal nitroglycerin. Normally the same absolute dose of buccal nitroglycerin is dissolved within 10 min compared to 0.8 mg of sublingual nitroglycerin. With both application forms the same plasma levels were reached. Plasma levels remained high for at least 60 min if the buccal tablet remains in place. Following sublingual nitroglycerin plasma concentration falls rapidly.

There is no question that buccal Synchron nitroglycerin is a rapid onset long-acting nitrate. Its pharmacokinetic-hemodynamic profile is comparable to an intravenous infusion of nitroglycerin [2, 4].

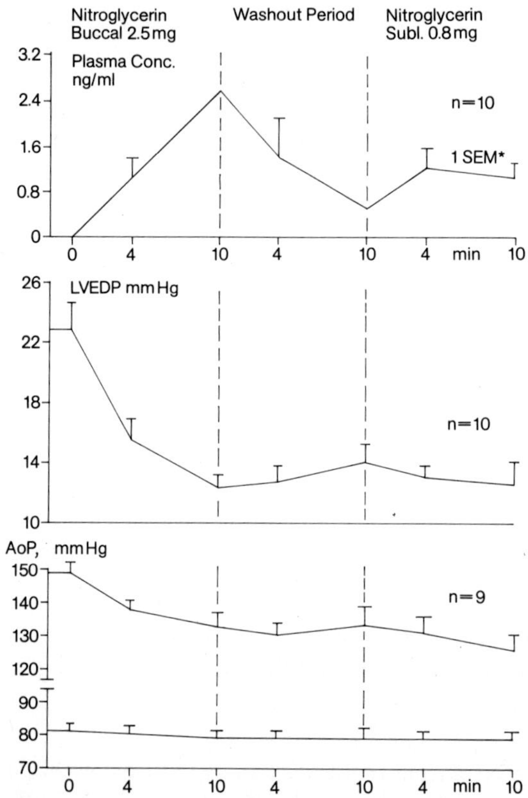

Fig. 7. Pharmacokinetic and pharmacodynamic data of the comparison between buccal and sublingual nitroglycerin: A washout period of 10 min was allowed between the two. Nitroglycerin plasma concentration increased within 10 min and a fall was observed during the washout phase. Following sublingual nitroglycerin a re-increase was observed. Left ventricular end-diastolic pressure dropped as well as systolic aortic pressure. During the washout period a slight re-increase occurred. The hemodynamic response to sublingual nitroglycerin was minimal due to the briefness of the washout period.

References

1 Armstrong, P.W.; Armstrong, J.A.; Marks, G.S.: Blood levels after sublingual nitroglycerin. Circulation *59:* 585 (1979).

2 Armstrong, P.W.; Armstrong, J.A.; Marks, G.S.: Pharmacokinetic-hemodynamic studies of intravenous nitroglycerin in congestive cardiac failure. Circulation *62:* 160 (1980).

3 Armstrong, P.W.; Armstrong, J.A.; Marks, G.S.: Pharmacokinetic-hemodynamic studies of nitroglycerin ointment in congestive heart failure. Am. J. Cardiol. *46:* 670 (1980).

4 Bussmann, W.-D.; Passek, D.; Seidel, W.; Kaltenbach, M.: Reduction of CK and CK-MB indexes of infarct size by intravenous nitroglycerin. Circulation *63:* 615 (1981).

W.-D. Bussmann, MD, Center of Internal Medicine, Department of Cardiology,
University Clinic of the Johann Wolfgang Goethe University,
D-6000 Frankfurt a.M. (FRG)

Discussion

Chairmen: *J. Abrams* and *H.J. Becker*

Davis: You were talking about dissolution; however, the release process is mainly one of diffusion through the gel created around the tablet. For instance we can recover tablets from an in vitro dissolution apparatus, the tablet is still intact, but there is no drug left in measuring the change in size of the tablet. It might be possible to recover a tablet where there was no drug remaining. It would be a better procedure if the amount of drug remaining in the tablet was assayed by chemical methods.

Bussmann: But nevertheless, as you can see from the blood levels, there was a relationship between the rest of the tablet and the plasma levels. But your opinion is that a tablet can stay at the same size and all the nitroglycerin is gone. Is that correct?

Davis: Yes, you will get some reduction in size as the gel erodes but a 40% reduction in the size of the tablet does not necessarily mean that you have lost the equivalent amount of drug.

Abrams: It raises very interesting questions, if one is a believer that nitroglycerin acts peripherally by reducing myocardial workload, then why pay attention to coronary arteries that are vasodilating, but I suspect that the vasodilation has some role in relieving angina.

Bussmann: Dr. *William Ganz* evaluated patients by pacing induced angina and then injected nitroglycerin intracoronarily. He couldn't observe a relief of angina. But I think we have to look again at this problem, since this mechanism we just spoke about – dilatation of the narrowed segment – may be important and a very crucial point for the action of nitroglycerin to relieve angina.

Reichek: It was of interest to me that at the termination of our outpatient trials, a substantial proportion of the patients chose to continue to use the buccal nitroglycerin in preference to oral agents and sublingual nitroglycerin that they had used previously. There are many patients who have relatively infrequent but predictable angina during their daily life. They find it helpful to have an agent that has immediate but lasting effects. This eliminates the need to take medication continually, which they regard as a great liability.

Davis: Figure 5 of my paper shows what happens when a volunteer moves the tablet from the cheek pouch and thereby alters the release rate. Thus, a patient should be able to slow up or speed up the release pattern by altering the dissolution process in the mouth.

Schor: It is a dicisive advantage to have a fast onset as well as prolonged activity because this gives greater flexibility in use of the tablet. Since the onset activity is comparable to that of a sublingual preparation the buccal tablet could be used to relieve an anginal attack or it could be used prophylactically for long-term use because of the prolonged effect. The patient then would not have to carry several preparations with him, but rather one that could do double duty.

Lichstein: You have to remember, though, that there is a double-edged sword to this; the higher the dose that you use the better it is for the prophylactic effect, but that gives you more problems with the immediate onset. The higher dose makes it more likely that you may get an immediate hypotensive effect, so that presents something of a problem.

Bussmann: Normally we put our patients with angina pectoris on a three times daily schedule, taking a tablet in the morning, noon and in the evening. Dr. *Reichek* proposed another approach: a tablet is used only if there is a need, and you take the tablet out if you don't need it anymore. This is a totally different approach to patient care. I think it's a good approach, but we also need a fixed dose frequency regimen.

Becker: Which blood level is needed to have a safe clinical effect? Can you give me an answer? Is it 0.2 or what?

Bussmann: 0.5 ng/ml is a good level. Using the buccal form levels in the range from 0.5 to 2.5 ng/ml are possible. This has nothing to do with the oral form with much lower levels. But I think with the buccal form, 0.5 to 1.0 ng/ml is sufficient. In our institution using isosorbide dinitrate in large doses the strategy is six times daily 20 or 40 mg. This is a heavy strategy for the compliance of our patients. With a buccal tablet, I think he needs only two or three tablets a day, so this is an advantage. Dr. *Reichek*, do you have any experience with patients having a buccal tablet in place at night? We all have patients waking up at 6.00 o'clock in the morning due to angina.

Erb: It looks from the data that we've seen that the therapeutic range that is being delivered by ointment, topical, which is delivering in a pretty high consistent rate is nearing 1–3 ng/ml, so 0.5 ng per ml upwards looks to us to be a therapeutic range. I would say that I always start thinking therapeutic at about 1 ng/ml.

Reichek: We do have some experience in a very limited number of patients. Our initial concern was safety. It appears to be safe and for patients that get nocturnal angina in the small hours of the morning, it appears to be effective on the basis of limited observations. I'm not sure whether the duration of effect will be sufficient to prevent the initial episode of angina that patients so commonly get on rising. But we've observed that because of the rapid onset, those individuals are able to have the medication at the bedside, take it immediately, and then they get a period of prophylaxis during that period of rising and washing which is very often the time when the patient with angina gets the first episode of symptoms during the day.

Schor: I'd just like to make a comment. The patient who doesn't get frequent anginal attacks or who doesn't want to take medication on a regular basis can, however, take the buccal tablet at the time of a stressful situation or when he knows he wants to undertake an activity that causes him angina. We call this acute prophylaxis. The patient will be protected by the nitroglycerin for a period of time, whether it be a 0.5, 1 or 2 h. When he's finished with that event or exercise or whatever stressful situation he can remove the tablet and discard it if he wants to.

Adv. Pharmacother., vol. 1, pp. 73–97 (Karger, Basel 1982)

Effect of Buccal Synchron Nitroglycerin on Pulmonary Artery Pressure at Rest and during Exercise

A Comparison with Sublingual Nitroglycerin in Patients with Coronary Artery Disease

A.-F. Langbehn[a], *H.W. Beurich*[a], *H. Leupold*[a], *R. Hoffmann*[a], *A. Sheikhzaden*[b], *R. Lohaus*[b]

[a] Rehabilitationszentrum Bad Segeberg, Bad Segeberg, FRG; [b] EDP and Biostatistics Department, Dr. Thiemann GmbH, Lünen, FRG

Introduction

As a short-acting nitrate nitroglycerin leads to direct relaxation of smooth muscle in the venous system. This systemic venodilation without significant alteration in total peripheral vascular resistance [*Mason and Braunwald,* 1965] results in decreased venous return, decreased pulmonary artery pressure, and decreased left ventricular end-diastolic pressure. In addition to the predominant venodilation, nitroglycerin may affect a modest decline in regional vascular resistance [*Mason* et al., 1980]. This hemodynamic change is probably the major cause for relief of acute myocardial ischemia and angina pectoris.

Since the pharmacological action of nitroglycerin is short, great efforts are being made to develop long-acting nitrate formulations [*Langbehn* et al., 1978], such as controlled-release nitroglycerin preparations.

The purpose of the present investigation is to study acute effects following buccal administration of different dosages of a controlled-release nitroglycerin formulation (buccal Synchron nitroglycerin).

Material and Methods

60 patients with ischemic heart disease and angina pectoris, their age ranging between 44 and 74 years (mean age 59 ± 8 years), were included in this controlled randomized comparative study. 47 patients (78%) were male and 13 (22%) female. Prior to the study all patients underwent a complete clinical examination, routine laboratory tests, and electrocardiographic examinations. All of them suffered from coronary artery disease demonstrated by electrocardiographic changes and/or positive exercise test results. 12 patients (20%) also had coronary angiograms revealing significant coronary artery disease. All patients had typical angina pectoris episodes for a period of 22 ± 10 months. The frequency of angina pectoris attacks was 4 ± 2/week. A positive response to sublingually administered nitroglycerin could be observed in all patients. 9 patients required concomitant digitalis therapy because of congestive heart failure.

The patients were randomly assigned to one of the following groups: group I was treated with 1.0 mg, group II with 2.5 mg, group III with 5.0 mg buccally administered Synchron nitroglycerin, and group IV, the control group, with 0.8 mg nitroglycerin administered sublingually.

Hemodynamic measurements were performed using a pulmonary artery catheter (Grandjean) introduced from the right basilic or the right saphenous vein. Exercise testing was done with a bicycle ergometer in recumbent position at work loads of 25, 50, 75, 100, and 125 W for 3-min periods.

Pulmonary artery pressures (systolic, diastolic, mean), heart rate, systemic blood pressure, and changes of the ST segment in the electrocardiogram were recorded before administration of the test drugs as well as 5, 15, 30, 60, 120 and 180 s after it during exercise. Exercise testing was performed 3, 30, and 180 min after application. Exercise was discontinued when the patient had angina pectoris symptoms with concomitant ST depression between 0.2 and 0.4 mV.

The above-described acute phase was preceded by a 1-week basic therapy phase with 2.6 mg orally administered Synchron nitroglycerin twice daily.

Statistical Analysis

In line with the aim of our study, the biostatistical evaluation concentrated on investigating the effect of four drug doses on our target variables during the acute dosing phase. Therefore, the intraindividual pre-/postdrug differences were examined with the paired t test for the three study phases. By adapting the significance level with the Bonferroni test, we allowed for the multiple character of the test hypothesis.

The homogeneity test of our four study groups at onset of our study was performed by the one-way analysis of variance or by the nonparametric H test by Kruskal-Wallis. The nonparametric data were checked using the χ^2-test.

Results

Homogeneity Tests

Comparing the study groups in respect of demographic and history data at the onset of our investigations did not reveal any statistically significant differences. During exercise testing at baseline (study onset) a few parameters were statistically significant in the analysis of variance (table I).

Table I. Statistically significant parameters at baseline (analysis of variance)

Parameter	Degrees of freedom	F value	p value
At 2 min exercise			
Diastolic pulmonary artery pressure	3/18	3.433	0.039
ST segment depression	3/18	4.085	0.022
At 3 min exercise			
ST segment depression	3/18	3.791	0.029
5 min after exercise stop			
Heart rate	3/32	4.159	0.014

Table II. Statistical significance for premedication data at onset of the acute phase

Parameter	Degrees of freedom	F value	p value
At rest			
ST segment depression	3/20	3.197	0.046
At exercise stop			
Relief of angina pectoris pain	3/22	5.846	0.004
Asymptomatic	3/22	3.777	0.025

The homogeneity test at the onset of the acute phase resulted in the statistical significances for premedication data shown in table II.

The interindividual differences between baseline values of the basic therapy phase and all other parameters of the acute phase were not significant.

Pulmonary Artery Pressure at Rest

The effect of the test agent on pulmonary artery pressure at rest in the early phase after application is documented in table III and in figure 1. The pulmonary artery pressure is measured six times during 180 s. As early as 30 s after application of any test drug, pressure values start falling and show a pronounced decrease after another 30 s. The strongest effect is observed after buccal administration of 2.5 mg Synchron nitroglycerin: after 5 s the pulmonary artery pressure starts falling, continues falling, and the systolic pressure fall is statistically significant ($p < 0.01$) 30 s after administration. The largest reduction is measured after 180 s with 5.6 mm Hg%. The same trend

Table III. Pulmonary artery pressure (mm Hg) after application at rest (mean values)

Time after administration, s	Nitroglycerin, mg				Comparison of study groups[1]	
	1.0 buccal	2.5 buccal	5.0 buccal	0.8 sublingual	degrees of freedom	F value[2]
Systolic pulmonary artery pressure						
0	22.9	23.2	23.5	22.5	3/48	0.082
5	23.0	21.8	20.1	23.8	3/28	0.409
15	24.0	20.6	20.8	24.8	3/28	0.816
30	22.0	19.2	22.6	21.0	3/33	0.666
60	20.1	18.6	20.6	20.0	3/50	0.345
120	20.6	18.8	19.3	19.0	3/46	0.260
180	20.0	17.6	18.3	17.3	3/52	0.745
Diastolic pulmonary artery pressure						
0	8.2	7.0	6.5	7.4	3/48	0.346
5	10.0	6.9	6.1	7.0	3/28	1.230
15	9.4	6.3	7.5	5.6	3/28	1.109
30	7.3	4.1	6.6	4.9	3/33	1.228
60	7.5	4.9	5.5	4.8	3/50	1.406
120	7.2	4.0	5.5	4.4	3/46	1.550
180	6.6	4.7	4.2	4.7	3/52	0.974
Mean pulmonary artery pressure						
0	14.5	13.6	12.9	14.1	3/48	0.270
5	15.3	12.8	12.1	14.3	3/28	0.551
15	15.6	12.0	12.8	13.1	3/28	0.650
30	13.7	10.5	12.9	11.6	3/33	0.973
60	13.2	11.1	11.2	11.4	3/50	0.690
120	13.3	10.4	11.3	10.8	3/46	1.029
180	12.4	10.5	10.0	10.1	3/52	0.951

[1] One-way analysis of variance.
[2] Not significant ($p > 0.05$).

is to be observed in diastolic and mean pulmonary artery pressures: the diastolic pressure is statistically significant after 60 s ($p < 0.05$), and the mean pressure decreases after 30 s ($p < 0.05$). After sublingual administration of 0.8 mg nitroglycerin, the pulmonary artery pressure values show a similar tendency, except for the initial phase of 15 s, during which the systolic pressure shows a minor increase; however, comparable values are achieved as late as 120 s. At no point of time could statistically significant differences be observed among the four study groups.

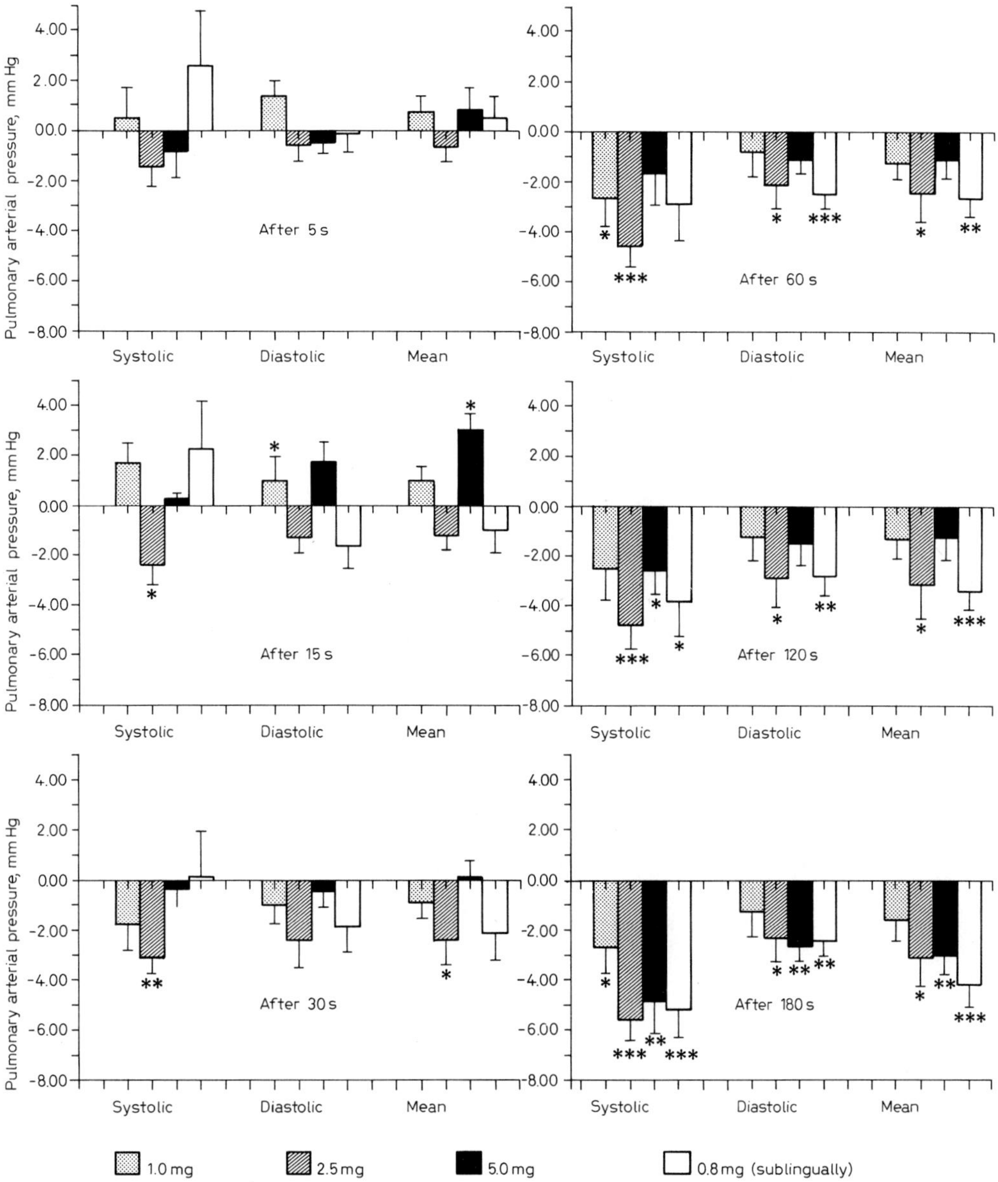

Fig. 1. Pulmonary arterial pressure early after administration. Mean differences to pre-values (mean values ± SD). $^{*}p < 0.05$; $^{**}p < 0.01$; $^{***}p < 0.001$.

Pulmonary Artery Pressure during Exercise

During the acute phase, exercise testing has been performed after measurements at rest 3, 30, and 180 min after application. Starting from a work load of 25 W, the work load has been increased by 25 W every 3 min up to a maximum well-tolerated load to be discontinued at any manifestation of symptoms.

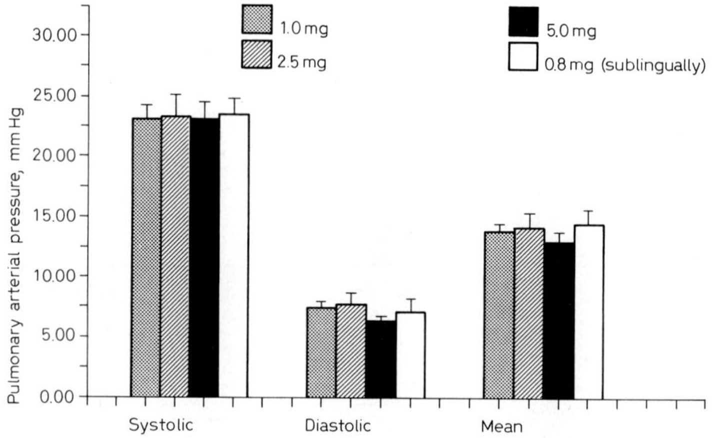

Fig. 2. Pulmonary arterial pressure. Resting values before load (mean values ± SD).

Table IV. Exercise testing: systolic pulmonary artery pressure (mm Hg) – mean values and standard deviation (SD)

	Group[1]	1st day (admission)		Acute phase (8th day)							
				before administration		3 min after administration		30 min after administration		180 min after administration	
		mean	SD	mean	SD	mean	SD	mean	SD	mean	SD
At rest	I	22.9	3.8	23.1	4.3	no data		15.3***	3.7	20.5**	4.7
	II	23.3	5.1	23.3	7.1			14.1***	3.4	19.0*	5.5
	III	24.4	5.4	23.1	5.3			15.4***	3.9	19.7*	3.9
	IV	23.3	7.1	23.5	5.1			17.8**	3.7	22.5	5.2
25 W	I	31.0	8.1	36.9	4.8	28.1	5.0	26.3***	5.1	31.3**	4.5
0 min	II	39.4	5.6	40.8	11.9	27.6***	7.6	24.0***	7.0	33.4*	9.6
	III	43.7	15.7	36.5	6.1	25.5***	6.8	26.3***	6.5	34.9	7.6
	IV	42.4	10.9	37.6	1.9	31.6*	9.9	29.4***	8.9	34.8	11.3

Table IV (continued)

	Group[1]	1st day (admission)		Acute phase (8th day)							
				before administration		3 min after administration		30 min after administration		180 min after administration	
		mean	SD	mean	SD	mean	SD	mean	SD	mean	SD
25 W	I	35.2	8.6	40.1	6.0	31.4***	6.0	28.5***	4.7	36.5	6.3
1 min	II	43.0	11.1	45.9	12.0	30.7***	8.9	28.1***	9.3	37.7**	11.6
	III	47.5	12.0	43.5	9.1	26.5***	6.7	26.2***	6.2	39.5**	8.1
	IV	51.3	16.0	45.2	12.5	30.7***	7.9	33.1***	8.2	40.9	12.1
25 W	I	38.2	8.3	43.1	6.3	31.5***	6.4	29.6***	5.6	38.9**	8.1
2 min	II	44.0	15.4	46.2	10.7	32.4***	9.3	29.3***	10.1	43.8**	14.1
	III	46.4	6.7	46.7	11.7	27.0***	7.1	27.1***	5.3	42.6	8.6
	IV	56.6	10.7	47.4	12.4	31.7***	8.1	35.6***	8.4	44.4	12.2
50 W	I	41.8	8.6	46.2	6.5	35.1***	7.8	31.0***	5.4	42.8	9.6
3 min	II	49.0	13.1	51.0	12.1	35.6***	9.6	32.0***	11.7	45.9	14.9
	III	53.1	12.2	49.7	11.5	29.3***	7.6	28.7***	5.5	44.8*	9.7
	IV	50.8	14.0	49.6	9.0	33.6***	7.3	37.8***	8.5	44.5	11.6
50 W	I	46.0	7.3	47.2	7.5	35.0***	7.5	33.7***	7.4	44.1	8.1
4 min	II	56.8	5.5	52.8	12.3	36.8***	10.8	34.1***	11.6	43.9*	13.8
	III	53.9	13.6	52.8	12.3	36.8***	10.8	34.1***	11.6	43.9	13.8
	IV	51.8	14.0	51.2	9.1	37.6***	9.6	39.2**	9.1	46.3	11.4
50 W	I	50.6	9.1	48.6	8.4	35.7**	9.1	33.0***	7.4	45.8	8.6
5 min	II	58.9	11.7	49.2	14.7	39.5*	11.4	33.9**	13.0	41.1	14.1
	III	51.5	12.4	47.1	8.5	33.3***	8.8	30.6***	6.3	44.9	12.1
	IV	48.2	12.8	51.8	10.4	38.0**	8.7	40.6*	10.5	45.3	12.7
75 W	I	44.0		51.1	8.0	35.3**	8.0	35.0**	7.3	47.9	8.8
6 min	II	65.8		47.3	12.3	35.7	11.1	28.3*	7.5	45.6	14.7
	III	0.0		48.3	10.3	34.3**	9.5	33.7**	6.9	45.2	7.0
	IV	54.0		53.2	9.7	39.1*	7.7	43.6	9.5	45.0	9.8
75 W	I	48.5	7.2	51.1		35.9**	7.5	37.6*	8.0	51.8	8.6
7 min	II	59.4	17.0	42.0		35.3	14.9	32.3	12.1	44.0	12.8
	III	50.3	11.3	43.0	10.4	30.0*	6.3	36.1	10.6	46.5	7.0
	IV	48.8	10.3	50.3	10.0	40.4	7.7	38.0	6.2	49.3	10.5
75 W	I	49.0		52.6		36.9**	8.2	39.1*	8.1	50.7	8.9
8 min	II	65.0		42.0		35.8	14.6	35.0	12.2	46.5	13.5
	III	40.0		46.0		30.0*	7.7	29.6	5.7	47.8	8.2
	IV	45.0		45.5		40.4	8.9	39.0	7.1	51.3	11.1

[1] I = 1.0 mg, II = 2.5 mg, III = 5.0 mg nitroglycerin buccally; IV = 0.8 mg nitroglycerin sublingually (controls).
* $p < 0.05$; ** $p < 0.01$; *** $p < 0.001$.

In figure 2, pulmonary artery pressure values at rest before exercise testing are demonstrated. The individual baseline values for the treatment groups are homogeneous. The pre- and postdrug pulmonary artery pressure values for the various work load increases are summarized in tables IV and V. During the 3-min postdrug exercise bout, the intraindividual pre-/post comparison based on the same work load increase showed a significant systolic reduction by approximately 20–40% and a significant diastolic pulmonary artery pressure reduction by approximately 25–50% up to a work load of 50 W/5 min in all four study groups. Under nitroglycerin administered buccally, the decreasing trend is confirmed even after 30 min up to 75 W work load compared with premeasurement values; by contrast, sublingually applied nitroglycerin gradually starts another increase in systolic pulmonary artery pressure during the 2nd min of exercise and is statistically significant at the 4th min. The trend of diastolic pressure during exercise is similar to the systolic one as was to be expected.

After 180 min, a marked increase in systolic pulmonary artery pressure is recorded compared with the 30-min data in all study groups. After buccally administered nitroglycerin, however, several statistically significant differences to premeasurement can be found up to the 4th min during exercise. Reviewing our diastolic measurements, only the two lower buccally administered nitroglycerin doses show statistically significant values, whereas the diastolic values of the other groups approach premedication values after 3 h.

Table V. Exercise testing: diastolic pulmonary artery pressure (mm Hg) – mean values and standard deviation (SD)

	Group[1]	1st day (admission)		Acute phase (8th day)							
				before administration		3 min after administration		30 min after administration		180 min after administration	
		mean	SD	mean	SD	mean	SD	mean	SD	mean	SD
At rest	I	7.7	3.1	7.4	2.1	no data		3.7***	2.1	5.9*	2.5
	II	11.0	15.3	7.7	3.4			3.5***	2.3	5.3*	2.4
	III	6.7	3.1	6.3	1.4			2.8***	2.4	6.5	2.7
	IV	7.3	4.0	7.1	4.2			5.5	4.0	6.2	2.9
25 W	I	13.3	5.9	14.3	3.9	9.6***	3.3	7.5***	2.3	10.5**	1.6
0 min	II	17.6	3.0	16.8	6.2	10.0***	4.6	7.8***	4.0	12.1*	5.4
	III	17.3	7.4	13.3	4.3	7.3***	3.1	7.1***	2.8	13.7	5.9
	IV	20.2	8.6	14.7	5.9	9.3***	3.9	11.2**	5.1	13.5	5.4

Table V (continued)

	Group[1]	1st day (admission)		Acute phase (8th day)							
				before administration		3 min after administration		30 min after administration		180 min after administration	
		mean	SD	mean	SD	mean	SD	mean	SD	mean	SD
25 W	I	16.4	7.6	15.9	4.4	11.2***	4.6	8.9***	2.6	13.7*	3.2
1 min	II	20.7	2.5	20.3	7.6	11.2***	5.8	9.2***	5.2	14.9*	6.8
	III	19.3	7.3	15.3	4.7	7.5***	3.2	7.4***	2.2	16.1	5.5
	IV	20.4	8.8	18.1	6.0	11.5***	5.3	12.8**	4.8	17.0	6.8
25 W	I	17.0	4.2	17.3	4.8	11.2***	3.7	9.4***	2.7	13.9**	3.9
2 min	II	22.7	4.2	20.6	6.4	11.9***	5.7	10.1***	5.1	15.7**	7.2
	III	17.0	7.1	17.8	7.1	7.9***	3.5	7.8***	2.3	18.7	6.2
	IV	25.4	5.4	19.7	6.3	12.0***	5.9	14.9**	5.2	18.8	7.4
50 W	I	20.3	4.8	19.6	5.0	12.4***	4.0	11.1***	3.7	15.9**	5.2
3 min	II	21.3	3.2	23.5	8.5	13.7***	6.3	12.4***	7.7	17.6**	7.1
	III	25.7	7.6	17.6	7.1	8.6***	3.5	8.6***	2.7	18.4	6.7
	IV	24.8	7.7	21.8	5.5	13.5***	4.3	16.1***	6.1	18.2	5.1
50 W	I	22.0	4.7	21.1	5.3	13.0***	3.8	12.4***	4.6	16.2**	4.5
4 min	II	24.6	10.2	24.1	9.2	14.7***	7.4	13.6***	8.0	17.6*	6.8
	III	25.2	8.1	17.1	5.4	9.2**	4.0	8.5***	2.6	17.1	7.9
	IV	22.7	7.5	21.9	6.1	18.2***	14.0	16.8*	6.4	20.1	6.7
50 W	I	23.7	6.8	21.3	6.2	14.1**	4.7	13.0**	4.7	17.6	4.8
5 min	II	23.6	3.8	21.2	10.6	13.6**	7.2	13.4**	8.3	16.6	6.9
	III	20.4	8.4	15.5	4.0	9.6**	4.3	8.7***	3.2	18.0	9.2
	IV	20.5	6.9	22.3	6.0	15.1***	6.3	17.0*	6.3	19.0	7.4
75 W	I	21.5		21.6	4.4	13.3**	4.8	12.7**	3.3	18.6	3.1
6 min	II	24.6		18.0	7.6	10.0*	5.8	9.2*	5.9	17.9	8.0
	III	0.0		16.5	3.3	11.5**	5.9	10.6**	3.6	18.5	4.0
	IV	24.0		23.6	7.8	16.1	5.6	18.8	6.1	19.6	4.7
75 W	I	21.0	4.7	22.4		14.4*	4.9	14.1*	4.2	20.4	4.3
7 min	II	23.0	5.9	13.0		11.8	7.1	11.5	6.6	17.8	8.7
	III	22.0	9.1	16.7	4.2	9.3*	4.1	11.4	4.6	16.5	4.1
	IV	21.3	8.5	21.0	9.6	15.7	5.8	15.5	4.9	21.8	7.7
75 W	I	24.8		24.6		14.4**	4.2	14.9*	4.7	20.1	4.7
8 min	II	27.0		13.0		11.8	7.1	12.5	6.8	18.5	8.2
	III	19.0		19.7		10.3*	5.8	9.4	3.6	15.3	6.7
	IV	15.0		18.5		17.0	5.7	18.8	5.9	23.3	6.4

[1] I = 1.0 mg, II = 2.5 mg, III = 5.0 mg nitroglycerin buccally; IV = 0.8 mg nitroglycerin sublingually (controls).
* $p < 0.05$; ** $p < 0.01$; *** $p < 0.001$.

ST Segment Depression

As we know, ST segment depression represents a parameter with a relatively wide interindividual variation. This is confirmed by the values at rest shown in figure 3. The mean values of study groups III and IV differ significantly before the acute phase. Tables VI and VII as well as figure 4 demon-

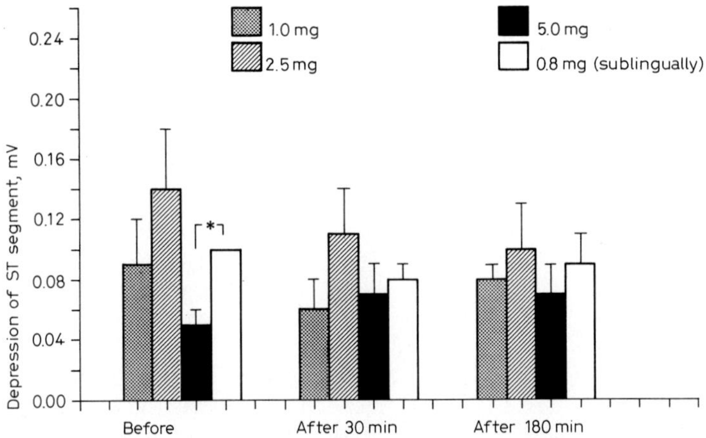

Fig. 3. Depression of ST segment. Resting values before load (mean values ± SD). *$p < 0.05$.

Table VI. Exercise testing: ST segment depression (mV) – mean values and standard deviation (SD)

	Group[1]	1st day (admission)		Acute phase (8th day)							
				before administration		3 min after administration		30 min after administration		180 min after administration	
		mean	SD	mean	SD	mean	SD	mean	SD	mean	SD
At rest	I	0.062	0.063	0.090	0.065	no data		0.060	0.042	0.075	0.029
	II	0.117	0.113	0.140	0.089			0.107	0.067	0.100	0.061
	III	0.070	0.027	0.050	0.027			0.067	0.029	0.067	0.029
	IV	0.108	0.049	0.100	0.0			0.080	0.027	0.090	0.042
25 W	I	0.050	0.071	0.057	0.065	0.037	0.055	0.030**	0.056	0.037*	0.061
0 min	II	0.067	0.098	0.083	0.084	0.040**	0.066	0.057	0.070	0.040**	0.017
	III	0.050	0.063	0.053	0.048	0.017**	0.024	0.020*	0.032	0.033	0.036
	IV	0.160	0.108	0.093	0.103	0.050**	0.065	0.047*	0.044	0.060	0.071

Table VI (continued)

	Group[1]	1st day (admission)		Acute phase (8th day)							
				before administration		3 min after administration		30 min after administration		180 min after administration	
		mean	SD	mean	SD	mean	SD	mean	SD	mean	SD
25 W 1 min	I	0.058	0.074	0.090	0.089	0.060	0.076	0.040**	0.057	0.067	0.108
	II	0.093	0.146	0.147	0.113	0.050***	0.071	0.071***	0.080	0.057***	0.068
	III	0.092	0.080	0.080	0.059	0.033**	0.036	0.023**	0.042	0.050**	0.053
	IV	0.214	0.146	0.143	0.128	0.073***	0.110	0.060***	0.063	0.110	0.117
25 W 2 min	I	0.083	0.082	0.100	0.092	0.070*	0.075	0.057**	0.068	0.057**	0.073
	II	0.050	0.077	0.150	0.114	0.063***	0.072	0.079***	0.085	0.083**	0.084
	III	0.110	0.089	0.117	0.092	0.047**	0.040	0.040**	0.043	0.063*	0.052
	IV	0.230	0.110	0.180	0.137	0.093***	0.132	0.083***	0.092	0.118**	0.128
50 W 3 min	I	0.083	0.068	0.127	0.081	0.103**	0.101	0.080***	0.084	0.079**	0.087
	II	0.150	0.141	0.175	0.123	0.090***	0.091	0.100***	0.094	0.100***	0.096
	III	0.217	0.093	0.146	0.092	0.073**	0.042	0.043***	0.042	0.137	0.099
	IV	0.317	0.076	0.200	0.138	0.089***	0.084	0.111**	0.100	0.146	0.157
50 W 4 min	I	0.115	0.080	0.169	0.107	0.104***	0.101	0.097***	0.092	0.100**	0.096
	II	0.187	0.140	0.200	0.139	0.107**	0.078	0.118***	0.097	0.086**	0.084
	III	0.211	0.134	0.155	0.112	0.079*	0.032	0.054**	0.048	0.115	0.103
	IV	0.212	0.126	0.178	0.094	0.072**	0.106	0.108*	0.082	0.133	0.166
50 W 5 min	I	0.177	0.099	0.150	0.085	0.100**	0.095	0.083**	0.069	0.121	0.089
	II	0.200	0.127	0.190	0.175	0.120	0.114	0.105*	0.109	0.081	0.084
	III	0.185	0.085	0.200	0.175	0.096*	0.050	0.061*	0.066	0.131*	0.122
	IV	0.200	0.130	0.175	0.080	0.090**	0.057	0.110	0.057	0.114	0.085
75 W 6 min	I	0.100	0.050	0.156	0.073	0.075**	0.065	0.072***	0.067	0.110	0.057
	II	0.026	0.210	0.275	0.166	0.075	0.027	0.075*	0.076	0.107**	0.093
	III	0.0		0.233	0.232	0.115	0.047	0.062	0.038	0.133	0.088
	IV	0.233		0.200	0.100	0.106*	0.077	0.150	0.085	0.158	0.107
75 W 7 min	I	0.158	0.086	0.171		0.087*	0.095	0.087**	0.095	0.137	0.069
	II	0.210	0.124	0.188		0.112	0.063	0.112	0.085	0.133	0.140
	III	0.175	0.050	0.133		0.075	0.029	0.087*	0.064	0.112	0.025
	IV	0.200	0.141	0.125		0.143	0.127	0.112	0.025	0.175	0.125
75 W 8 min	I	0.150		0.193		0.106*	0.129	0.100**	0.096	0.143*	0.073
	II	0.350		0.100		0.112	0.063	0.125	0.096	0.162	0.170
	III	0.200		0.167	0.029	0.112	0.063	0.060*	0.055	0.137	0.048
	IV	0.100		0.167	0.104	0.150	0.141	0.150	0.058	0.187	0.111

[1] I = 1.0 mg, II = 2.5 mg, III = 5.0 mg nitroglycerin buccally; IV = 0.8 mg nitroglycerin sublingually (controls).
* $p < 0.05$; ** $p < 0.01$; *** $p < 0.001$.

Table VII. ST segment depression during/after maximum exercise tolerance (mV) – mean values and standard deviation (SD)

	Group[1]	1st day (admission)		Acute phase (8th day)							
				before administration		3 min after administration		30 min after administration		180 min after administration	
		mean	SD	mean	SD	mean	SD	mean	SD	mean	SD
At discon-	I	0.218	0.067	0.237	0.095	0.163***	0.122	0.153***	0.079	0.200*	0.100
tinuation	II	0.273	0.151	0.247	0.133	0.143**	0.102	0.136***	0.097	0.177**	0.094
of exercise	III	0.223	0.096	0.250	0.138	0.117***	0.049	0.103***	0.061	0.197	0.088
	IV	0.280	0.098	0.283	0.106	0.200**	0.127	0.210**	0.078	0.263	0.137
1 min	I	0.131	0.066	0.123	0.096	0.093*	0.080	0.107	0.084	0.123	0.100
after	II	0.125	0.089	0.153	0.142	0.089*	0.084	0.093*	0.083	0.107*	0.092
disconti-	III	0.145	0.079	0.120	0.096	0.080*	0.049	0.077*	0.062	0.083*	0.052
nuation	IV	0.215	0.103	0.163	0.126	0.113**	0.092	0.110*	0.060	0.127	0.102
2 min	I	0.107	0.070	0.113	0.101	0.083**	0.088	0.097	0.090	0.117	0.099
after	II	0.163	0.137	0.140	0.144	0.079*	0.078	0.093	0.090	0.113	0.090
disconti-	III	0.104	0.063	0.110	0.083	0.073	0.050	0.067**	0.056	0.067*	0.041
nuation	IV	0.164	0.112	0.137	0.113	0.087**	0.077	0.077*	0.062	0.113	0.092
3 min	I	0.100	0.059	0.093	0.084	0.077	0.088	0.093	0.092	0.097	0.097
after	II	0.142	0.196	0.143	0.157	0.070*	0.068	0.064**	0.066	0.100	0.089
disconti-	III	0.106	0.062	0.093	0.059	0.057*	0.037	0.060**	0.043	0.057**	0.053
nuation	IV	0.135	0.091	0.123	0.115	0.070*	0.059	0.060*	0.057	0.097	0.083
5 min	I	0.050	0.041	0.073	0.080	0.053*	0.079	0.067	0.082	0.073	0.075
after	II	0.137	0.172	0.100	0.118	0.062	0.074	0.057	0.062	0.054*	0.072
disconti-	III	0.070	0.071	0.063	0.052	0.043	0.037	0.043	0.042	0.043*	0.042
nuation	IV	0.075	0.072	0.083	0.088	0.043*	0.050	0.040	0.043	0.073	0.073
7 min	I	0.033	0.029	0.053	0.055	0.043	0.068	0.047	0.061	0.057	0.078
after	II	0.050	0.076	0.073	0.100	0.054	0.066	0.050	0.071	0.053	0.081
disconti-	III	0.067	0.061	0.043	0.050	0.040	0.039	0.027	0.032	0.017*	0.036
nuation	IV	0.080	0.076	0.063	0.072	0.030*	0.041	0.037*	0.044	0.050	0.057

[1] I = 1.0 mg, II = 2.5 mg, III = 5.0 mg nitroglycerin buccally; IV = 0.8 mg nitroglycerin sublingually (controls).
* $p < 0.05$; ** $p < 0.01$; *** $p < 0.001$.

strate that in all study groups the exercise-induced ST segment depression is already significantly reduced ($p < 0.01$) 3 min after application at maximum exercise tolerance. The same holds good for all groups 30 min after drug application. After 180 min, however, significant values are only achieved by the two lower buccally administered nitroglycerin doses, whereas after sublingual administration of nitroglycerin no significant reduction can be shown.

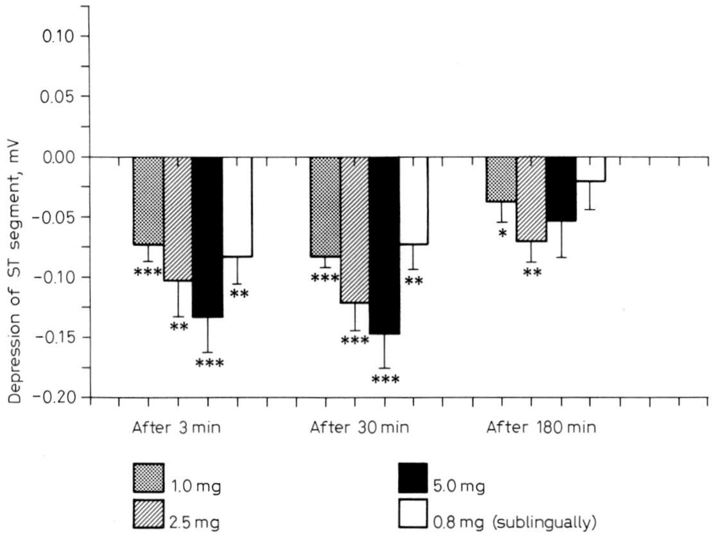

Fig. 4. Depression of ST segment at maximum load. Mean differences to prevalues (mean values ± SD). * $p < 0.05$; ** $p < 0.01$; *** $p < 0.001$.

Exercise Tolerance

Exercise tolerance (fig. 5, table VIII) as well as the duration of exercise (fig. 6, table IX) are also significantly increased 3 min after application in all study groups ($p < 0.05$). The maximum increases during exercise are observed 30 min after buccal administration of 5 mg ($p < 0.001$) and 3 h after buccal administration of 2.5 mg nitroglycerin ($p < 0.05$). After sublingual administration of nitroglycerin, the improvement is most pronounced at 3 min and thereafter reduces steadily.

The increased exercise tolerance of our patients was also reflected in the prolonged duration of exercise to the occurrence of angina pectoris symptoms quantifiable 30 min after buccal administration of 2.5 mg nitroglycerin ($p < 0.05$) as well as in the shortened period of relief until the patient is asymptomatic (table X).

Major criteria leading to a discontinuation of exercise in the predrug phase were severe ECG changes as well as increasing angina pectoris symptoms and severe fatigue (table XI). A positive effect of 2.5 or 5 mg buccally administered Synchron nitroglycerin on ECG changes with resulting discontinuation of exercise is reflected in a reduction of the frequency of discontinuation by 50–60% 30 min after administration of nitroglycerin.

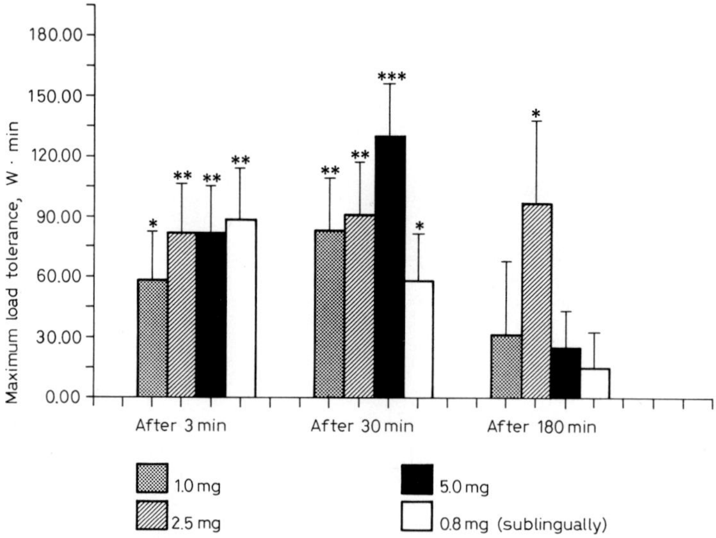

Fig. 5. Maximum load tolerance. Mean differences to prevalues (mean values ± SD). $^{*}p < 0.05$; $^{**}p < 0.01$; $^{***}p < 0.001$.

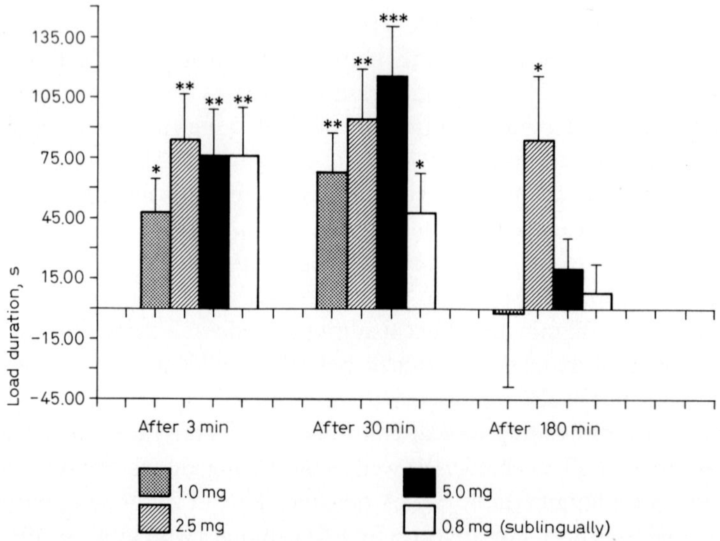

Fig. 6. Load duration. Mean differences to prevalues (mean values ± SD). $^{*}p < 0.05$; $^{**}p < 0.01$; $^{***}p < 0.001$.

Table VIII. Exercise testing: exercise tolerance (W/min)

	1st day (admission)	Acute phase (8th day)			
		before adminis-tration	3 min after adminis-tration	30 min after adminis-tration	180 min after adminis-tration
1.0 mg nitroglycerin administered buccally (group I)					
Mean values	300	305	363*	388**	336
Standard deviation	185	195	215	219	186
Minimum	50	25	100	150	25
Maximum	725	725	725	725	725
2.5 mg nitroglycerin administered buccally (group II)					
Mean value	293	213	295**	309**	310*
Standard deviation	215	258	247	250	282
Minimum	25	25	100	150	50
Maximum	850	1,100	1,100	1,100	1,100
5.0 mg nitroglycerin administered buccally (group III)					
Mean value	237	213	295**	343***	238
Standard deviation	112	133	134	136	158
Minimum	100	50	100	100	100
Maximum	425	425	625	625	625
0.8 mg nitroglycerin administered sublingually (group IV, controls)					
Mean value	228	248	337**	307*	263
Standard deviation	186	242	258	242	278
Minimum	25	50	50	50	25
Maximum	625	975	1,100	975	1,100

* $p < 0.05$; ** $p < 0.01$; *** $p < 0.001$.

Blood Pressure, Heart Rate, and Oxygen Consumption

At the end of exercise testing, systolic and diastolic blood pressures show a marked decline. The most pronounced differences from predrug measurements are found after buccal application of 2.5 or 5 mg Synchron nitroglycerin with up to 17/7 or 19/6 mm Hg and can still be demonstrated 7 min after the 30-min exercise testing was terminated ($p < 0.01$). After application of all test drugs, the heart rate is only moderately affected during low to moderate

Table IX. Exercise testing: duration of exercise (s)

	1st day (admission)	Acute phase (8th day)			
		before adminis-tration	3 min after adminis-tration	30 min after adminis-tration	180 min after adminis-tration
1.0 mg nitroglycerin administered buccally (group I)					
Mean value	328	424	472*	492**	422
Standard deviation	180	167	163	159	169
Minimum	180	120	240	300	120
Maximum	720	720	720	720	720
2.5 mg nitroglycerin administered buccally (group II)					
Mean value	313	328	412**	424**	412*
Standard deviation	153	181	166	166	203
Minimum	120	120	240	300	180
Maximum	600	900	900	900	900
5.0 mg nitroglycerin administered buccally (group III)					
Mean value	280	352	428**	468***	372
Standard deviation	95	126	108	107	135
Minimum	120	180	240	240	240
Maximum	480	540	660	660	660
0.8 mg nitroglycerin administered sublingually (group IV, controls)					
Mean value	256	368	444**	416*	376
Standard deviation	112	180	181	172	205
Minimum	120	180	180	180	120
Maximum	480	840	900	840	900

* $p < 0.05$; ** $p < 0.01$; *** $p < 0.001$.

work load of exercise testing up to 30 min and is reduced to lower values on average by 3–9 beats/min after 180 min. As shown in figure 7 the heart rate is increased after 3 min during maximum work load by 4–9 beats/min in all four study groups ($p < 0.05$). A similar situation can be observed after 30 min. After 3 h, the heart rate has returned to normal baseline values. Tables XII–XVII show the normalization trend of systolic and diastolic blood pressures as well as of the heart rate during the first 7 min after exercise.

Table X. Exercise testing: angina pectoris pain during exercise (mean values)

Parameter	Group[1]	1st day (admission)	8th day			
			before adminis-tration	3 min after adminis-tration	30 min after adminis-tration	180 min after adminis-tration
Angina pectoris symptoms during exercise (frequency)	I	6	5	2	1	6
	II	8	8	4	5	7
	III	8	6	3	2	2
	IV	9	9	6	6	5
Time until manifestation, s	I	175	252	270	420	330
	II	233	203	285	316*	249
	III	203	210	380	450	270
	IV	160	262	340	253	244
Time until relief, s	I	83	45	60	60	75
	II	120	146	135	108	94
	III	113	80	80	90	120
	IV	120	75	73	83	84
Time until asymptomatic, s	I	130	128	120	120	130
	II	180	214	120	156*	154
	III	173	130	140	150	180
	IV	173	127	132	156	120

[1] I = 1.0 mg, II = 2.5 mg; III = 5.0 mg nitroglycerin buccally; IV = 0.8 mg nitroglycerin sublingually (controls).
* $p < 0.05$.

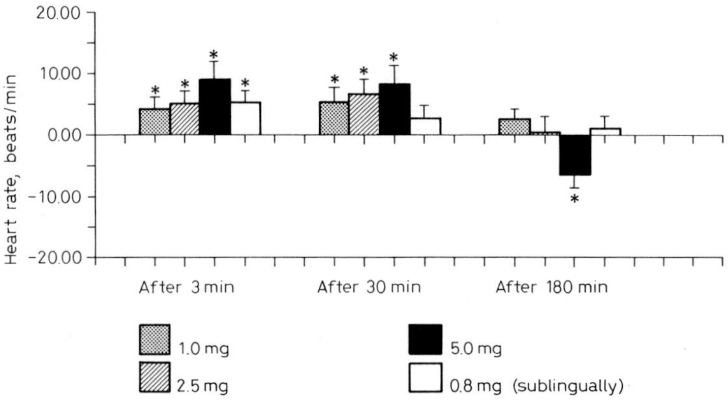

Fig. 7. Heart rate at maximum load. Mean differences to prevalues (mean values ± SD). * $p < 0.05$.

Table XI. Exercise testing: frequency of major criteria for discontinuation

Parameter	Group[1]	1st day (admission)	8th day before administration	8th day 3 min after administration	8th day 30 min after administration	8th day 180 min after administration
Angina pectoris symptoms	I	7	5	2	1	6
	II	8	8	4	5	7
	III	8	6	3	2	2
	IV	8	8	5	5	6
Severe dyspnea	I	1	3	2	4	2
	II	6	1	1	3	2
	III	5	3	–	3	3
	IV	1	6	3	4	5
Dizziness	I	–	–	1	1	–
	II	–	1	–	–	–
	III	–	–	–	–	–
	IV	–	1	–	–	–
Severe fatigue	I	5	8	10	9	8
	II	2	6	9	9	6
	III	5	7	9	10	6
	IV	5	7	10	11	9
Heart rate, maximum tolerance	I	1	–	–	–	–
	II	1	–	–	1	–
	III	–	–	–	–	–
	IV	–	–	–	–	–
Severe ECG changes	I	15	15	8	10	10
	II	14	14	9	7	12
	III	12	15	6	6	13
	IV	14	14	8	11	12

[1] I = 1.0 mg, II = 2.5 mg, III = 5.0 mg nitroglycerin buccally; IV = 0.8 mg nitroglycerin sublingually (controls).

Table XII. Exercise testing: systolic blood pressure (mm Hg) before and during exercise (mean values)

	Group[1]	1st day (admission)	8th day before administration	8th day 3 min after administration	8th day 30 min after administration	8th day 180 min after administration
At rest	I	136	130	no data	120*	128
	II	142	138		122**	127*
	III	138	134		116**	133
	IV	147	136		126**	140
Onset of exercise	I	153	136	134	124**	135
	II	147	141	132**	129*	137
	III	146	140	131*	126*	145
	IV	164	147	135***	135**	145
After 2 min (work load 25 W)	I	147	151	145	142*	149
	II	167	153	149	147*	150
	III	158	151	144*	143	156
	IV	177	159	154	154	156
After 5 min (work load 50 W)	I	167	159	149	152	155
	II	165	170	164	157	160
	III	168	163	161	155	156
	IV	175	165	165	168	155
After 8 min (work load 75 W)	I	183	170	166	174	168
	II	210	175	179	175	174
	III	155	183	170	166	170
	IV	–	173	169	164	169

[1] I = 1.0 mg, II = 2.5 mg, III = 5.0 mg nitroglycerin buccally; IV = 0.8 mg nitroglycerin sublingually (controls).
* $p < 0.05$; ** $p < 0.01$; *** $p < 0.001$.

Table XIII. Exercise testing: systolic blood pressure (mm Hg) after exercise (mean values)

Time after exercise, min	Group[1]	1st day (admission)	8th day			
			before administration	3 min after administration	30 min after administration	180 min after administration
1	I	157	153	147	140*	152
	II	155	152	140**	135**	152
	III	163	152	138***	138***	148
	IV	160	154	153	155	154
2	I	150	142	140	133*	139
	II	159	144	130**	128**	143
	III	149	145	128***	124***	141
	IV	152	149	144	144	147
3	I	138	134	131	126*	131
	II	153	137	122***	120***	136
	III	146	139	121***	121***	131*
	IV	158	142	135	137	143
5	I	128	128	125	121*	125
	II	148	131	121**	116***	131
	III	135	129	119*	116***	126
	IV	150	138	128*	130	136
7	I	120	125	119*	119**	124
	II	141	130	118**	113***	130
	III	135	129	116**	114**	125
	IV	136	133	126*	129	133

[1] I = 1.0 mg, II = 2.5 mg, III = 5.0 mg nitroglycerin buccally; IV = 0.8 mg nitroglycerin sublingually (controls).
* $p < 0.05$; ** $p < 0.01$; *** $p < 0.001$.

Table XIV. Exercise testing: diastolic blood pressure (mm Hg) before and during exercise (mean values)

	Group[1]	1st day (admission)	8th day			
			before adminis-tration	3 min after adminis-tration	30 min after adminis-tration	180 min after adminis-tration
At rest	I	82	82	no data	81	84
	II	89	83		78**	78*
	III	88	82		77	86
	IV	87	85		83	87
Onset of exercise	I	87	88	87	82*	88
	II	93	86	84	83*	86
	III	92	88	86	82*	90
	IV	95	87	90	85	90
After 2 min (work load 25 W)	I	88	90	92	88	92
	II	104	93	92	89*	88
	III	99	92	91	90	96
	IV	98	93	94	92	95
After 5 min (work load 50 W)	I	97	97	91*	92	97
	II	99	105	98	92	94
	III	101	94	96	93	97
	IV	99	97	97	99	94
After 8 min (work load 75 W)	I	100	101	96	97	99
	II	100	100	98	96	95
	III	105	97	100	98	100
	IV	–	108	101	100	105

[1] I = 1.0 mg, II = 2.5 mg, III = 5.0 mg nitroglycerin buccally; IV = 0.8 mg nitroglycerin sublingually (controls).
* $p < 0.05$; ** $p < 0.01$.

Table XV. Exercise testing: diastolic blood pressure (mm Hg) after exercise (mean values)

Time after exercise, min	Group[1]	1st day (admission)	8th day before adminis-tration	8th day 3 min after adminis-tration	8th day 30 min after adminis-tration	8th day 180 min after adminis-tration
1	I	95	92	88	83**	89
	II	92	90	85*	83***	88
	III	98	87	86	85	92
	IV	98	88	87	88	91
2	I	89	86	84	84	85
	II	94	87	80**	80***	83
	III	89	86	81***	80**	87
	IV	91	87	85	86	89
3	I	85	84	83	83	82
	II	92	83	79	78**	84
	III	93	83	79*	80*	84
	IV	92	84	84	84	87
5	I	83	81	82	82	81
	II	89	82	80	77**	82
	III	88	82	79	77**	83
	IV	94	83	82	84	86
7	I	80	80	81	80	80
	II	91	81	77	80	80
	III	87	82	77*	76**	83
	IV	83	81	81	83	86

[1] I = 1.0 mg, II = 2.5 mg, III = 5.0 mg nitroglycerin buccally; IV = 0.8 mg nitroglycerin sublingually (controls).
* $p < 0.05$; ** $p < 0.01$; *** $p < 0.001$.

Table XVI. Exercise testing: heart rate (beats/min) before and during exercise (mean values)

	Group[1]	1st day (admission)	8th day before adminis-tration	8th day 3 min after adminis-tration	8th day 30 min after adminis-tration	8th day 180 min after adminis-tration
At rest	I	74	78	no data	87	72*
	II	71	77		91**	68*
	III	74	81		90*	69***
	IV	71	74		77	67*
Onset of exercise	I	87	98	99	98	90***
	II	101	94	94	94	88*
	III	87	93	97**	95	88***
	IV	89	92	94	92	87
After 2 min (work load 25 W)	I	104	103	104	102	95***
	II	107	102	100	103	93***
	III	92	98	101	99	91***
	IV	85	100	99	97	91*
After 5 min (work load 50 W)	I	112	110	113	112	107
	II	103	106	115	109	100*
	III	106	105	112	109	97*
	IV	111	107	106	107	107
After 8 min (work load 75 W)	I	128	123	126	127	122
	II	115	94	119	110	104
	III	121	115	131	125*	111
	IV	110	122	118	121	126

[1] I = 1.0 mg, II = 2.5 mg, III = 5.0 mg nitroglycerin buccally; IV = 0.8 mg nitroglycerin sublingually (controls).
* $p < 0.05$; ** $p < 0.01$; *** $p < 0.001$.

Table XVII. Exercise testing: heart rate (beats/min) after exercise (mean values)

Time after exercise, min	Group[1]	1st day (admission)	8th day			
			before adminis-tration	3 min after adminis-tration	30 min after adminis-tration	180 min after adminis-tration
1	I	96	93	102*	104**	93
	II	85	87	98***	99*	85
	III	89	87	107***	103***	81*
	IV	88	86	97**	91*	82
2	I	86	87	96**	98***	85
	II	81	80	91***	94*	79
	III	83	84	105***	96***	77**
	IV	78	81	87*	88*	79
3	I	80	84	93***	94***	83
	II	71	81	93***	91**	78
	III	84	84	102**	95***	73***
	IV	78	80	86*	83	76
5	I	100	81	91**	93***	80
	II	78	76	88***	87**	77
	III	75	80	98***	91**	74*
	IV	78	76	83**	80*	74
7	I	88	80	90**	89***	78
	II	73	76	87***	87***	76
	III	80	81	96***	94***	75*
	IV	73	76	82*	79	72

[1] I = 1.0 mg, II = 2.5 mg, III = 5.0 mg nitroglycerin buccally; IV = 0.8 mg nitroglycerin sublingually (controls).
* $p < 0.05$; ** $p < 0.01$; *** $p < 0.001$.

Table XVIII. Exercise testing: mixed venous saturation (%) before and during exercise (mean values)

	Group[1]	1st day (admission)	8th day			
			before adminis-tration	3 min after adminis-tration	30 min after adminis-tration	180 min after adminis-tration
At rest	I	74	75	no data	72**	73*
	II	75	77		70***	72***
	III	75	77		70***	73***
	IV	75	76		72***	74**
Onset of exercise	I	69	65	65	64	66
	II	70	68	66	62***	64**
	III	68	67	63*	61***	65
	IV	65	68	65	66	66
After 2 min (work load 25 W)	I	61	58	58	57	56*
	II	61	59	57	54**	55*
	III	59	60	57*	54***	56**
	IV	50	58	58	58	56
After 5 min (work load 50 W)	I	50	54	52	53	51**
	II	53	54	49*	47	48
	III	56	57	48*	48*	53
	IV	53	55	56	54*	53**
After 8 min (work load 75 W)	I	47	48	49	48	46
	II	56	52	48	48	45
	III	46	55	53	51	50
	IV	46	55	53	52	53

[1] I = 1.0 mg, II = 2.5 mg, III = 5.0 mg nitroglycerin buccally; IV = 0.8 mg nitroglycerin sublingually (controls).
* $p < 0.05$; ** $p < 0.01$; *** $p < 0.001$.

The exercise-dependent mixed venous oxygen saturation in pulmonary artery (table XVIII) was reduced after all doses of buccally administered nitroglycerin in contrast to the effect of sublingually applied nitroglycerin. 3 min after buccal administration of 5 mg nitroglycerin, the mixed venous oxygen saturation in pulmonary artery were reduced ($p < 0.05$); this effect becomes more marked, and after 30 min ($p < 0.001$) it can be compared to the results after buccal administration of 2.5 mg Synchron nitroglycerin. After 3 h a normalization trend can be recognized resulting in alternating statistical findings.

Side Effects

The recorded adverse effects and concomitant symptoms are statistically summarized in table XIX. 5 of 7 patients complained of a heavy sensation or headaches of various degrees of severity. A relation to the test drug was assessed as 'probable' in 2 of those cases and as 'certain' in 2 other ones. Clinical and laboratory examinations did not show any pathological changes during our study.

Table XIX. Casuistics of side effects and concomitant symptoms

Number of patients	Group[1]	Time after administration min	Symptom/comment	Causal relationship
8	I	3	moderate malaise	certain
42	I	3	moderate headache	certain
10	II	3	moderate dizziness	
25	III	3	severe headache	probable
43	III	3	moderately heavy sensation	probable
43	III	30	headache	probable
51	IV	3	moderate gastric symptoms severe headache	possible certain

[1] I = 1.0 mg, II = 2.5 mg, III = 5.0 mg nitroglycerin buccally; IV = 0.8 mg nitroglycerin sublingually (controls).

Discussion and Conclusion

The antianginal effect of short-acting nitroglycerin has been well known since described by *Brunton* [1892]. The basic pharmacological action of these compounds consists of the relaxation of vascular, predominantly venous smooth muscle [*Chon and Gorling,* 1974; *Mason and Braunwald,* 1965]. The vasodilating effect of nitrates on larger coronary arteries has also been demonstrated [*Likaff* et al., 1964]. The effectivity seems to be due to a reduction in mechanical activity and oxygen requirement of the myocardium with subsequent reduction in ventricular wall tension [*Mason* et al., 1980; *Mason and Braunwald,* 1965] and left ventricular end-diastolic pressure. In addition to the effects on cardiac hemodynamics, these compounds also have a beneficial effect on myocardial blood flow and redistribution of coronary flow into the ischemic area [*Bache* et al., 1979]. Nitroglycerin given sublingually is the drug of choice for acute treatment of anginal attacks, but there is also a need for long-acting, controlled-release nitrate preparations such as the Synchron form to be administered buccally.

In the past the effectivity of long-acting nitrates has been the subject of controversy [*Needleman* et al., 1972]. Consequently, the acute action as well as the long-term effects of a new controlled-release formulation, such as buccally administered Synchron nitroglycerin, have to be investigated intensively and carefully in human pharmacological studies in order to establish beyond any doubt the proof of efficacy.

The present controlled study shows that buccally administered Synchron nitroglycerin leads to immediate hemodynamic and clinical effects. These are well documented by the reduction in pulmonary artery pressure values at rest and during exercise, the improvement of ST segment depression, the increase in exercise tolerance, and the reduction in oxygen consumption. These effects last several hours at least. Although the hemodynamic and angina-relieving effects of nitrates are most marked when patients are sitting or standing [*Leceraf,* 1971], the effects of buccally administered Synchron nitroglycerin were found to be present despite the supine position of the patients necessary for this investigation. The best effect was achieved with the dosage of 2.5 mg Synchron nitroglycerin administered buccally.

We conclude that buccally applied Synchron nitroglycerin has the same effects as nitroglycerin administered sublingually during the acute phase of treatment; however, its hemodynamic and clinical effects persist over a minimum time of 180 min.

References

Bache, R.J.; Ball, R.M.; Cobb, F.R.; Rembert, J.C.; Greenfield, J.C.: Effects of nitroglycerin on transmural myocardial blood flour in the unanesthetized dog. J. clin. Invest. *59:* 1219 (1979).

Brunton, T.L.: On the use of nitrite of amyl in angina pectoris. Lancet *ii:* 97 (1892).

Chon, P.P.; Gorling, R.: Physiologic and clinical actions of nitroglycerin. Med. Clin N. Am. *58:* 407 (1974).

Langbehn, A.-F.; Haase, W.; Klempien, E.J.: Wirkungsdauer zweier Isosorbiddinitratretard-präparate bei Koronarinsuffizienz. Cardiol. Bull. *16:* 97 (1978).

Leceraf, H.: Influences of body position on exercise tolerance, heart rate, blood pressure, and respiration in coronary insufficiency. Br. Heart J. *33:* 78 (1971).

Likoff, W.; Kasporian, H.; Lehman, J.S.; Segal, B.L.: Evaluation of 'coronary vasodilatator' by coronary angiography. Am. J. Cardiol. *13:* 7 (1964).

Mason, D.T.; Awan, A.N.; De Maria, A.N.; Lee, G.; Amsterdam, E.A.: Cardiocirculatory effects of nitrates in the treatment of clinical congestive heart failure; in Rudolph, Schrey, Nitrate II, p. 206 (Urban & Schwarzenberg, München 1980).

Mason, D.T.; Braunwald, E.: The effects of nitroglycerin and amylnitrate on arterial and venous tone in the human forearm. Circulation *32:* 755 (1965).

Muller, O.; Rovik, R.: Hemodynamic consequences of coronary heart disease with aberration during anginal pain and the effect of the nitroglycerin. Br. Heart J. *20:* 302 (1958).

Needleman, P.; Lancy, S.; Johnson, E.M.: Organic nitrates. Relationship between biotransformation and regional angina pectoris therapy. J. pharmac. exp. Ther. *181:* 489 (1972).

A.-F. Langbehn, MD, Rehabilitationszentrum Bad Segeberg, Kurpark,
D-2360 Bad Segeberg (FRG)

Discussion

Chairmen: *U. Gleichmann, N. Reichek*

Bussmann: You also used the high dose of the buccal tablet, 5 mg? We made some experience with this high dose. In 1 patient we observed a marked drop in blood pressure and an increase in heart rate. I heard from other groups that there are side effects. How many patients did you treat with 5 mg? You also showed that ST segment depression was less influenced by the 5-mg preparation, is that correct?

Langbehn: The side effects were less impressive in our population. We did not have to interrupt the investigation in a single case. Each group included 15 patients. The best results were achieved in group II with 2.5 mg buccally administered nitroglycerin, but the effect of 5.0 mg was not as impressive. The reasons for this action of the 5.0-mg nitroglycerin preparation are not quite clear. I believe that the bioavailability of this preparation might have an influence.

Erb: Using digital plethysmography, we have seen at least once, and I believe twice, an instance where higher doses of orally administered nitrate actually produced a smaller response. I do not know what that means. When it first happened we thought that it was artifactual. It was not related to formulation.

Reichek: Since the issue of adverse responses to the 5-mg preparation has been brought up, I think it is an important problem we had at the onset when we thought, based on the data that have been presented, that the 5-mg dosage would be clinically very useful. We had several experiences of hypotension. This was basically a supine study, so the absence of these adverse effects may not mean that they could not occur in clinical practice for those same individuals. Our own solution for the moment has been to use a very cautious progressive dose-titration, starting all patients with the 1-mg size. This has worked very successfully. I think it may be necessary to use some such approach in developing strategies for the clinical use of this agent.

Adv. Pharmacother., vol. 1, pp. 98–100 (Karger, Basel 1982)

Acute Effect of Buccal Synchron Nitroglycerin on Pacer-Induced Angina pectoris and Left Ventricular Enddiastolic Pressure

D. Kaiser, W. Tegen, A.-F. Langbehn, M. Hoppe
Rehabilitationszentrum, Bad Segeberg, FRG

The quick relief of effort angina pectoris in patients with coronary heart disease by buccal application of Synchron nitroglycerin could be confirmed in our clinic. To document this, we studied the effect of buccal Synchron nitroglycerin in a dosage of 2.5 mg on left ventricular enddiastolic pressure in pacer-induced tachycardia and recorded the time until angina disappeared.

7 patients, 4 male and 3 female, with coronary heart disease were studied. The average age of the group was 55 years (range 43–66). All patients had previously suffered transmural infarction. The coronary angiogram showed 2-vessel disease in 6 patients and 3-vessel disease in 1 patient. The ejection fraction was normal in all cases. The study was done during diagnostical left heart catheterization with informed consent of the patients.

Pressure measurements were taken with a pigtail catheter in the left ventricle. A bipolar pacing catheter was placed in the right atrium. The patients had received no medication for at least 2 days prior to study.

As figure 1 shows, atrial pacing was commenced at a rate of 15% above the basic spontaneous heart rate for 1 min and was increased by 20 beats every 2 min until angina occurred (method according to *Grüntzig* [1]). 15 s after onset of angina the patient received a buccal placebo. 15 s after the substance was given the rate of pacing was again reduced to the initial paced heart rate. After a recovery time of 10 min we repeated the same stimulation program, this time giving buccal Synchron nitroglycerin in a dosage of 2.5 mg.

We started with a mean paced heart rate of 84/min and reached angina level at a mean paced heart rate of 141/min. LV enddiastolic and LV systolic pressure were measured at the end of the first minute of stimulation and over a period of 30 s after administration of the substance. When the placebo was given, the enddiastolic pressure increased from 10.6 to 18.5 mm Hg after 15 s and was 15.6 mm Hg after 30 s. The corresponding data after nitroglycerin were 15.09 and 12.35 mm Hg, respectively.

The probability of statistical significance of the difference was calculated by the Student's t-test for paired data. The difference between the placebo effect and the nitroglycerin effect, 30 s after administration, was significant at the 0.05 confidence level. The LV systolic pressure did not differ significantly. In table I, no significant time difference was found for the disappearance of angina. 1 patient had to be excluded because he suffered angina

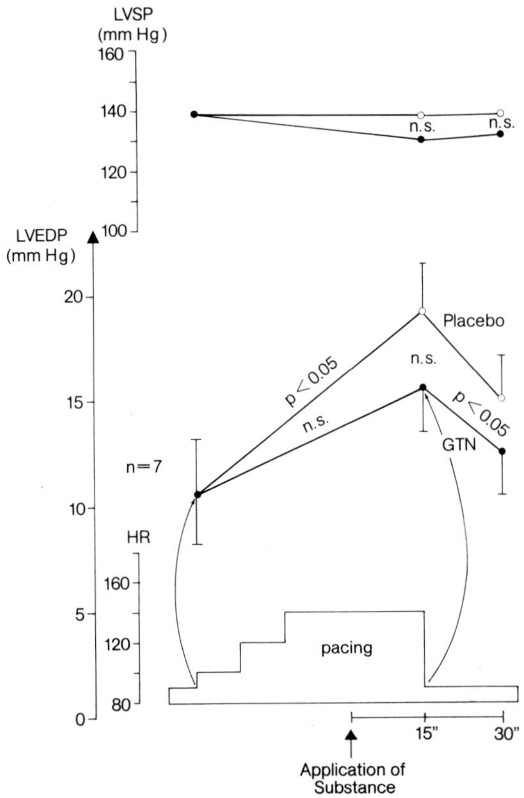

Fig. 1. Systolic (LVSP) and enddiastolic left ventricular pressure (LVEDP) during the pacing-induced changes in heart rate (HR) with buccal application of placebo or 2.5 mg Synchron nitroglycerin (GTN) (n = 6).

Table I. Effect of buccal Synchron nitroglycerin vs placebo on duration of pacer-induced angina in coronary patients

Patient No.	Placebo duration, s	Nitroglycerin duration, s
1	49	60
2	60	45
3	50	50
4	56	51
5	52	54
6	100	60
Mean	61.1	52.1
±SD	19.4	4.9

only during the first stimulation period. Therefore, I have data only for 6 patients. The results support the assumption of rapid resorption of Synchron nitroglycerin, applied in buccal form.

References

1 Grüntzig, A.: Wirkungseintritt des Isosorbiddinitratsprays. Nitrate II, p.403 (Urban & Schwarzenberg, München 1980).

2 Ganz, W.; Marcus, H.S.: Failure of intracoronary nitroglycerin to alleviate pacing-induced angina. Circulation *46:* 880 (1972).

D. Kaiser, MD, Rehabilitationszentrum, Kurhausstrasse 81,
D-2360 Bad Segeberg (FRG)

Discussion

Chairmen: *U. Gleichmann* and *N. Reichek*

Reichek: Dr. *Kaiser,* do you have any similar information about sublingual nitroglycerin? One of the questions that always comes up is whether in fact one could demonstrate efficacy of sublingual nitroglycerin in shortening duration of angina and, if so, with what kinds of study design. It's far from clear to me that this has really been done in a satisfactory way and one of the things I wonder about your protocol is whether it would demonstrate that sublingual nitroglycerin shortened the duration of angina.

Kaiser: That's right. Our results, I think, show that this study design is not very appropriate for demonstrating the duration of angina. But the effect on enddiastolic pressure was pronounced though I am not able to tell whether in another population this effect will be as pronounced or more or even less pronounced.

Adv. Pharmacother., vol. 1, pp. 101–115 (Karger, Basel 1982)

Effect of Buccally Administered Synchron Nitroglycerin on Pulmonary Artery Pressure

A Comparison with Sublingually Administered Nitroglycerin in Patients with Coronary Heart Disease

H. Ohlmeier, H.M. Mertens, H. Mannebach, U. Gleichmann

Gollwitzer-Meier-Institut, Klinik für Herz- und Kreislauferkrankungen, Bad Oeynhausen, FRG

Introduction

Pulmonary artery pressure at rest and during exercise is a reliable parameter of left ventricular dysfunction in patients with coronary heart disease. The antianginal effect of nitrates results from a reduction in pulmonary artery pressure during exercise due to a reduction in preload and afterload or venous pooling in patients with ischemia-induced left ventricular dysfunction.

The study was designed to compare potency and duration of action of 0.8 mg nitroglycerin administered sublingually and buccally administered Synchron nitroglycerin in two doses (1.0 and 2.5 mg), using as a parameter the reduction in pulmonary artery pressure at rest and during exercise in patients with coronary heart disease and left ventricular dysfunction.

Material and Methods

The study comprised 45 patients with coronary heart disease demonstrated by coronary arteriography in 42 cases. All patients showed exercise-induced angina pectoris with a pathological ECG during exercise. In most patients, left ventricular dysfunction was measured with a flotation catheter during exercise spirometry; a mean pulmonary artery pressure above 30 mm Hg during exercise was taken as abnormal. In this single-blind study, three groups of 15 patients each received 1.0 or 2.5 mg Synchron nitroglycerin buccally or 0.8 mg nitroglycerin sublingually in a randomized sequence after having given their informed consent.

These test groups were comparable in age, coronary heart disease, and exercise-induced left ventricular dysfunction (table I). Any negative or positive inotropic agents were discontinued prior to the study. All examinations were done at the same time of day.

Table I. Patient data of test drug groups

	Nitroglycerin sublingually	Controlled-Release nitroglycerin	
	0.8 mg	1.0 mg	2.5 mg
n	15	15	15
Sex ratio, m/f	14/1	14/1	14/1
Age, years (mean ± SD)	51.2 ± 6.9	52.4 ± 5.8	49.7 ± 7.6
Age range, years	40–65	43–62	37–67
1 Vessel occluded	5	5	2
2 Vessels occluded	4	3	3
3 Vessels occluded	6	6	8

The pulmonary artery pressure was measured by means of a flotation catheter in a recumbent position at rest, during volume load, and bicycle exercise testing at minute intervals. The work load was increased at 25-watt stages every minute.

At a mean pulmonary artery pressure of at least 30 mm Hg, the test agent was administered and exercise continued for another 3 min at a constant work load. This was followed by measurements at rest 5 min after application and during exercise with the individual work load 30, 60, 120 (15 patients) and 180 min after application of the test substance. Bipolar ECG monitoring was done during all exercise bouts and side-effects as well as angina pectoris data recorded.

Prior to exercise the cardiac output at rest was determined according to the Fick principle in 30 of the 45 patients, assuming a 95% artery oxygen saturation. The statistical analysis was performed using the t test, significance was assumed at the 5% level.

Results

Since the severity of coronary heart disease differed in the various test groups due to randomization, the three groups had to be subdivided according to the exercise tolerance, i.e., individual work load achieved at a minimum mean pulmonary artery pressure of 30 mm Hg. The subdivided individual results are first shown in comparison to heart rate and pulmonary artery pressure and then summarized in the three test agent groups. This seems possible because exercise testing was pressure oriented, i.e., all patients were tested to a mean pulmonary artery pressure of at least 30 mm Hg, the level at which the various test agents were compared.

In the group where 0.8 mg nitroglycerin were administered sublingually, 9 patients exercised to a work load of 25 W, 4 patients to 50 and 2 to 75 W.

Table II. Heart rate (beats/min) at rest and during exercise before and after application of nitroglycerin (mean ± SD)

Group	Nitro-glycerin mg	Rest	Predrug exercise	Exercise after drug administration		
				30 min	60 min	180 min
Maximum work load 25 W	0.8	77 ± 12	107 ± 8	104 ± 13	101 ± 14	103 ± 13
	1.0	69 ± 6	93 ± 7	93 ± 8	92 ± 11	91 ± 11
	2.5	70 ± 6	103 ± 11	94 ± 8	95 ± 6	97 ± 9
Maximum work load 50 W	0.8	74 ± 10	111 ± 4	112 ± 3	111 ± 6	112 ± 4
	1.0	80 ± 9	111 ± 17	109 ± 15	108 ± 14	109 ± 16
	2.5	69 ± 10	119 ± 20	123 ± 22	120 ± 21	119 ± 25
Maximum work load 75 W	0.8	67 ± 5	113 ± 11	112 ± 6	105 ± 7	106 ± 0
	1.0	78 ± 14	116 ± 4	123 ± 5	121 ± 4	119 ± 5
	2.5	71 ± 10	117 ± 15	127 ± 13	123 ± 14	119 ± 14

Table III. Effect of nitroglycerin at rest and during exercise on heart rate, systolic, diastolic, and mean pulmonary artery pressure (PAP; mean ± SD)

All patients	Nitro-glycerin mg	Rest	Predrug exercise	Exercise after drug administration		
				30 min	60 min	180 min
Heart rate beats, min	0.8	74 ± 11	109 ± 8	107 ± 11	104 ± 12	106 ± 11
	1.0	75 ± 10	105 ± 14	106 ± 15	105 ± 16	104 ± 17
	2.5	70 ± 8	113 ± 17	114 ± 21	114 ± 19	112 ± 20
PAP syst., mm Hg	0.8	25 ± 8	50 ± 7	43 ± 6	44 ± 6	53 ± 9
	1.0	27 ± 10	49 ± 11	41 ± 11	41 ± 12	46 ± 10
	2.5	24 ± 7	51 ± 9	33 ± 7	36 ± 8	44 ± 11
PAP diast., mm Hg	0.8	12 ± 4	26 ± 5	21 ± 5	22 ± 5	25 ± 6
	1.0	11 ± 6	25 ± 4	20 ± 5	19 ± 6	21 ± 4
	2.5	11 ± 4	27 ± 8	15 ± 6	16 ± 6	20 ± 7
Mean PAP, mm Hg	0.8	19 ± 4	39 ± 5	32 ± 5	33 ± 6	39 ± 7
	1.0	18 ± 8	37 ± 8	30 ± 8	29 ± 9	34 ± 8
	2.5	16 ± 6	40 ± 7	24 ± 6	25 ± 7	33 ± 9

In the group, which received 1.0 mg Synchron nitroglycerin buccally, 6 patients exercised to a work load of 25 W, 5 to 50, and 4 patients to 75 W, and after buccal application of 2.5 mg Synchron nitroglycerin 5 patients exercised to a work load of 25 W, 6 to 50, and 4 patients to 75 W. The results of the two groups which received Synchron nitroglycerin buccally are comparable, while those of the group which received 0.8 mg nitroglycerin sublingually had more patients at 25-watt work load and fewer at 75 W, though the severity of coronary heart disease in terms of number of occluded vessels is comparable with the other two groups.

Heart Rate

There were no statistically significant differences or a definite tendency in heart rate either between the individual groups or during the time course of 3 h. Significant differences at the 5% level could be demonstrated only between the groups which received 0.8 mg nitroglycerin sublingually or 1.0 mg Synchron nitroglycerin buccally in the subgroup results of 25 W work load during predrug exercise and in those of 75 W during exercise 60 min after application (table II). But the analysis of the three drug groups without considering the subgroups by work load did not result in any significant differences (table III, fig. 1).

Cardiac Output

The reduction in resting cardiac output did not show any significant differences in the various groups or during the 3-hour time course (fig. 2). However, during the time course a definite tendency to lowering of cardiac output emerges. This might be caused by the effect of the prolonged resting period making it particularly difficult to interpret the 3-hour data.

Acute Action

Figure 3 demonstrates the percentage changes in mean pulmonary artery pressure under steady state exercise conditions during the first 3 min after drug application. In the 1st min, all three groups showed a further increase in mean pulmonary artery pressure reflecting an increase in ischemia-induced left ventricular dysfunction. During the next 2 min there is a pronounced decrease in mean pulmonary artery pressure despite exercise continuation, particularly in patients who received 0.8 mg nitroglycerin sublingually and 2.5 mg Synchron nitroglycerin buccally. Due to considerable variation resulting from varying severity in coronary heart disease and different exercise tolerance, the differences in pulmonary artery pressure after acute dosing are not statistically significant. But the tendency suggests that the effect of 0.8 mg nitroglycerin sublingually and that of 2.5 mg Synchron nitroglycerin buccally are more pronounced than that of 1.0 mg Synchron nitroglycerin administered buccally.

1
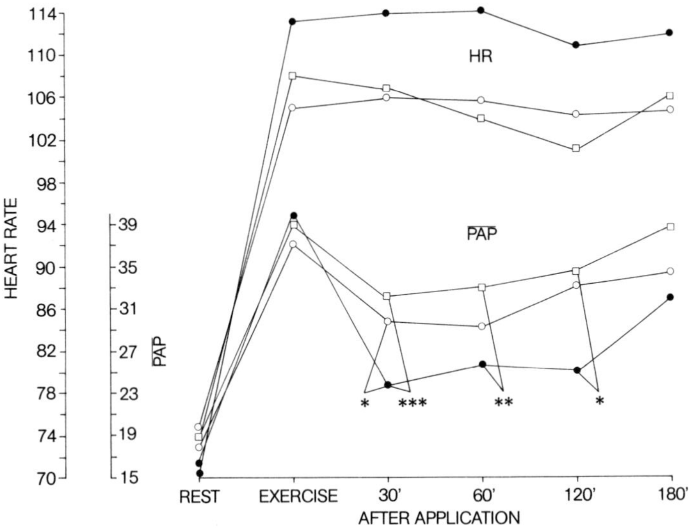

2
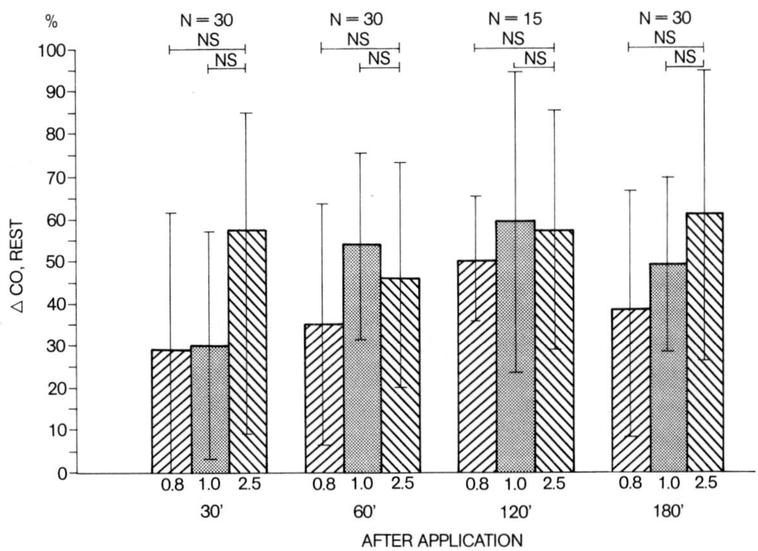

Fig. 1. Mean heart rate (HR, beats/min) and mean pulmonary artery pressure ($\overline{PAP}$, mm Hg) at rest and during exercise before and after application of nitroglycerin. ● = 2.5 mg nitroglycerin buccally (n = 15); □ = 0.8 mg nitroglycerin sublingually (n = 15); ○ = 1.0 mg nitroglycerin buccally (n = 15). $^{*}p < 0.05$; $^{**}p < 0.01$; $^{***}p < 0.001$.

Fig. 2. Percent reduction of resting cardiac index (CI, $1/min/m^2$) after application of 0.8, 1.0, or 2.5 mg nitroglycerin (mean ± SD).

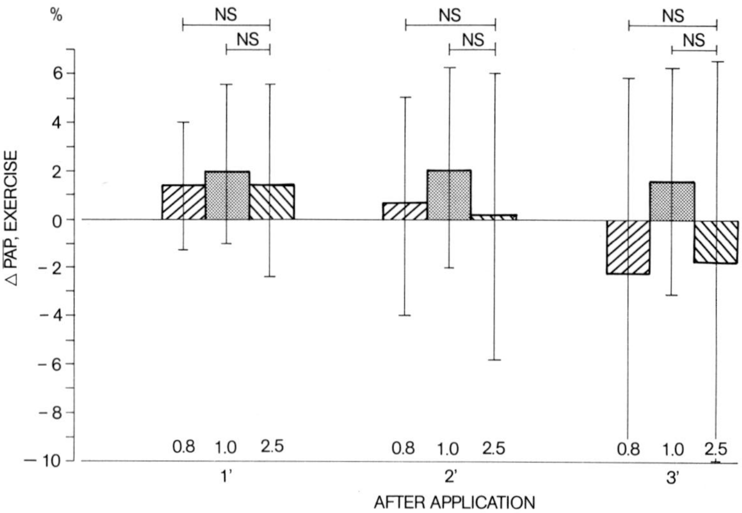

Fig. 3. Change in mean pulmonary artery pressure ($\overline{PAP}$, mm Hg) as percentage of baseline during the first 3 min after application of 0.8, 1.0, or 2.5 mg nitroglycerin under steady state conditions (mean ± SD).

Figure 4 shows mean pulmonary artery pressure values prior to drug application as well as those values for the 30-min resting phase after application measured at 5-min intervals. Corresponding to the pressure curve in the first 3 min after application, the reduction in pressure is nearly parallel after 0.8 mg nitroglycerin sublingually and after 2.5 mg Synchron nitroglycerin administered buccally, whereas 5 min after buccal application of 1.0 mg Synchron nitroglycerin the mean pulmonary artery pressure was still elevated compared to baseline values. The resulting reduction in pressure is less marked in the group with 1.0 mg Synchron nitroglycerin buccally than after the higher dose and after 0.8 mg nitroglycerin administered sublingually. 15 min after sublingual application of 0.8 mg nitroglycerin the maximum of action is achieved in this group in terms of reduction in mean pulmonary artery pressure at rest. During the next 10 min this group shows a reincrease in mean pulmonary artery pressure values whereas after buccal administration of 2.5 mg Synchron nitroglycerin the mean pulmonary artery pressures at rest continue to decline, resulting in statistically significant differences between the two groups after 20 min. 25 min after buccal application of 1.0 mg Synchron nitroglycerin a slight increase in mean pulmonary artery pressure at rest can be observed as well, thus also leading to significant pres-

4

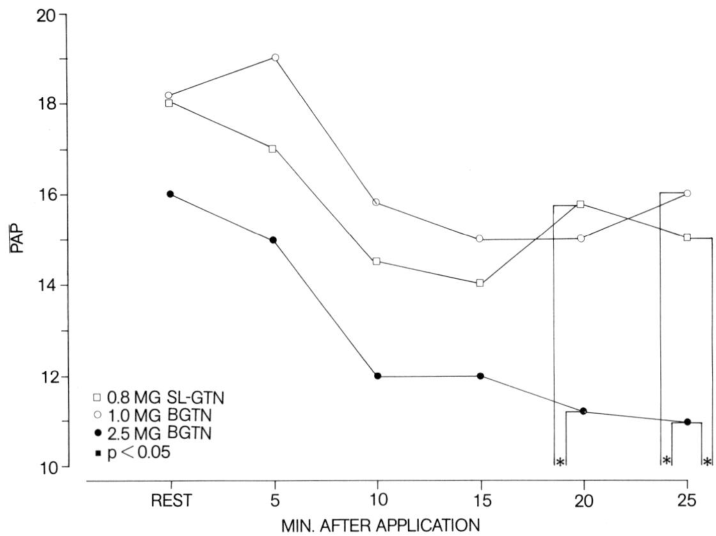

5

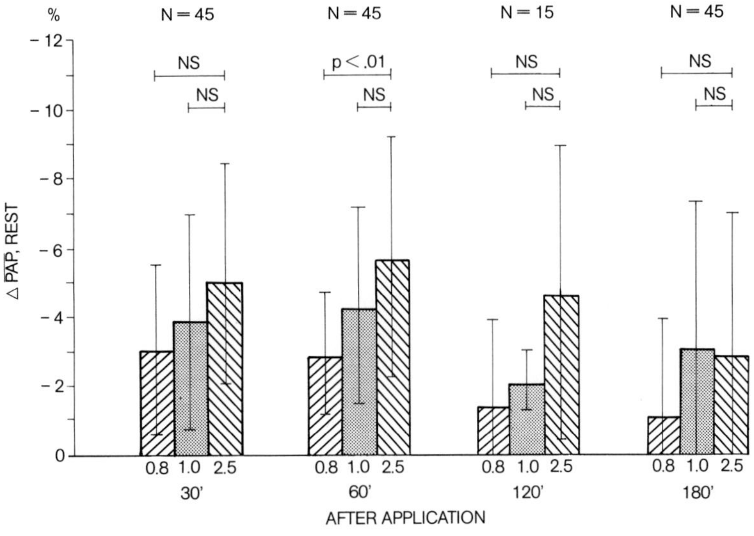

Fig. 4. Mean values of resting pulmonary artery mean pressure ($\overline{PAP}$, mm Hg) before and 25 min after application of nitroglycerin. *p < 0.05. ○ = 1.0 mg nitroglycerin buccally; □ = 0.8 mg nitroglycerin sublingually; ● = 2.5 mg nitroglycerin buccally.

Fig. 5. Mean values of resting pulmonary artery pressure ($\overline{PAP}$, mm Hg) after application of 0.8, 1.0, or 2.5 mg nitroglycerin (mean ± SD).

sure differences compared with the group which received 2.5 mg Synchron nitroglycerin buccally.

Pulmonary Artery Pressure at Rest

Figure 5 shows the effect of the three test drugs on mean pulmonary artery pressure at rest during a time course of 3 h. There is a relatively mild effect on mean resting pulmonary artery pressure that is most pronounced during the 1st h after application. After 60 min the effect of 2.5 mg Synchron nitroglycerin buccally is significantly higher than that of 0.8 mg sublingually administered nitroglycerin given the earlier maximum of action after sublingual nitroglycerin. The data at 120 min do not reveal any significant difference because of the low number of patients and the great variation, but the effect of 2.5 mg Synchron nitroglycerin administered buccally seems clearly more pronounced than that of the two other test preparations. After 180 min even these values are considerably influenced by the prolonged resting period.

Pulmonary Artery Pressure during Exercise

Tables IV–VI show the effect of the three nitroglycerin preparations on systolic, diastolic and mean pulmonary artery pressure during exercise at 30, 60, and 180 min after application, subdivided into exercise tolerance at 25, 50, and 75 W. Deriving from comparable predrug exercise values, the systolic pulmonary artery pressure values are significantly different at 25 W in the

Table IV. Systolic pulmonary artery pressure (mm Hg) at rest and during exercise before and after application of nitroglycerin (mean ± SD)

Group	Nitroglycerin mg	Rest	Predrug exercise	Exercise after drug administration		
				30 min	60 min	180 min
Maximum work load 25 W	0.8	28 ± 5	51 ± 5	44 ± 7	44 ± 8	51 ± 10
	1.0	35 ± 9	55 ± 14	48 ± 12	48 ± 13	52 ± 13
	2.5	29 ± 8	54 ± 13	33 ± 10	35 ± 12	44 ± 16
Maximum work load 50 W	0.8	26 ± 4	48 ± 7	40 ± 4	45 ± 5	55 ± 9
	1.0	25 ± 5	48 ± 5	39 ± 5	36 ± 6	44 ± 5
	2.5	23 ± 8	46 ± 3	34 ± 6	36 ± 7	43 ± 10
Maximum work load 75 W	0.8	15 ± 17	45 ± 11	40 ± 9	44 ± 8	60 ± 0
	1.0	19 ± 8	42 ± 6	34 ± 10	35 ± 12	41 ± 8
	2.5	22 ± 4	51 ± 9	32 ± 5	35 ± 5	48 ± 7

two groups which received 0.8 mg nitroglycerin sublingually and 2.5 mg nitroglycerin buccally given the earlier maximum of action for nitroglycerin sublingually. At a later point of time during exercise the pressure values after buccal administration of 2.5 mg Synchron nitroglycerin continue to be markedly lower than in the two other groups, but the difference is no longer statistically significant. The 50-watt work load subgroup shows statistically significant differences at the 5% level between 0.8 mg nitroglycerin sublingually

Table V. Diastolic pulmonary artery pressure (mm Hg) at rest and during exercise before and after application of nitroglycerin (mean ± SD)

Group	Nitro-glycerin mg	Rest	Predrug exercise	Exercise after drug administration		
				30 min	60 min	180 min
Maximum work load 25 W	0.8	12 ± 4	27 ± 5	21 ± 6	20 ± 4	24 ± 6
	1.0	15 ± 7	26 ± 6	22 ± 6	23 ± 7	24 ± 6
	2.5	15 ± 4	30 ± 8	16 ± 7	17 ± 6	23 ± 9
Maximum work load 50 W	0.8	13 ± 4	26 ± 5	21 ± 6	23 ± 7	27 ± 6
	1.0	9 ± 3	24 ± 4	18 ± 5	16 ± 5	20 ± 5
	2.5	9 ± 4	26 ± 6	18 ± 6	17 ± 8	21 ± 9
Maximum work load 75 W	0.8	9 ± 5	25 ± 1	22 ± 4	26 ± 6	27 ± 0
	1.0	8 ± 3	24 ± 3	17 ± 3	17 ± 1	23 ± 1
	2.5	8 ± 3	24 ± 11	10 ± 4	13 ± 4	19 ± 4

Table VI. Mean pulmonary artery pressure (mm Hg) at rest and during exercise before and after application of nitroglycerin (mean ± SD)

Group	Nitro-glycerin mg	Rest	Predrug exercise	Exercise after drug administration		
				30 min	60 min	180 min
Maximum work load 25 W	0.8	19 ± 4	41 ± 4	33 ± 6	32 ± 7	37 ± 9
	1.0	24 ± 9	40 ± 11	34 ± 10	35 ± 10	37 ± 11
	2.5	20 ± 7	43 ± 12	25 ± 8	26 ± 9	34 ± 12
Maximum work load 50 W	0.8	19 ± 3	38 ± 5	31 ± 5	35 ± 4	41 ± 3
	1.0	15 ± 4	36 ± 4	28 ± 5	26 ± 5	32 ± 5
	2.5	15 ± 5	38 ± 2	26 ± 5	26 ± 6	30 ± 8
Maximum work load 75 W	0.8	18 ± 0	36 ± 5	32 ± 3	36 ± 1	42 ± 0
	1.0	13 ± 4	34 ± 5	25 ± 4	26 ± 5	31 ± 3
	2.5	13 ± 1	38 ± 6	20 ± 6	24 ± 8	34 ± 7

and 1.0 mg Synchron nitroglycerin buccally after 60 and 180 min. Equivalent significant differences cannot be demonstrated for 0.8 mg nitroglycerin sublingually and 2.5 mg Synchron nitroglycerin administered buccally due to high variation, despite comparable mean pressure values. The same resasons (high variation, low number of patients) apply to the subgroup of 75 W work load where no significant differences in systolic pulmonary artery pressure during exercise could be detected.

The differences in diastolic pulmonary artery pressure are only statistically significant in the subgroup of 75 W, 30 and 60 min after application. 30 and 60 min after buccal application of 2.5 mg Synchron nitroglycerin, the diastolic pulmonary artery pressures are significantly lower than after sublingual application of 0.8 mg nitroglycerin and also lower than after buccal administration of 1.0 mg nitroglycerin, corresponding to the markedly different data at rest for the acute action 25 min after application. At 60 min the difference between 1.0 mg nitroglycerin buccally and 0.8 mg nitroglycerin sublingually is also statistically different, as can be expected from the prolonged effect of the Synchron formulation.

30 min after buccal application of 2.5 mg Synchron nitroglycerin at 25 W work load, the mean pulmonary artery pressure, as reference parameter for the left ventricular end-diastolic pressure, is significantly lower ($p < 0.05$) under exercise than after sublingual administration of 0.8 mg nitroglycerin. 60 and 180 min after application there are statistically significant differences ($p < 0.05$) between 2.5 or 1.0 mg Synchron nitroglycerin administered buccally and 0.8 mg nitroglycerin administered sublingually. This may be explained by the relatively lower mean pulmonary artery pressure at rest though the predrug pressures during exercise were comparable. At 75 W work load the pressure values are only significantly different between 0.8 mg nitroglycerin sublingually and 1.0 mg Synchron nitroglycerin buccally 60 min after application. The pressure values after buccal administration of 2.5 mg Synchron nitroglycerin are lower than after administration of 1.0 mg, but the pronounced variation does not allow statistical significance.

Disregarding exercise tolerance to ischemia-induced left ventricular dysfunction and summarizing the data for the three test drug groups individually, we arrive at a clearer picture (table III). Resting as well as exercise pressure prior to medication are comparable in all three groups. Systolic, diastolic, and mean pulmonary artery pressure values are significantly lowered ($p < 0.01$) 30 and 60 min after buccal application of 2.5 mg Synchron nitroglycerin as compared to the group wich received 0.8 mg nitroglycerin sublingually. 30 min after medication, the reduction in mean pulmonary artery pressure is significant at the 0.1% level. 180 min after buccal application of 2.5 mg Synchron nitroglycerin, the systolic pulmonary artery pressure during exercise is significantly lower than after nitroglycerin administered sublingually ($p < 0.05$). Moreover, 30 min after buccal application of 2.5 mg Synchron nitroglycerin, systolic and mean pulmonary artery pressures during exercise are significantly lower ($p < 0.05$) than after 1.0 mg (fig. 1). Even 120 min after buccal application of 2.5 mg Synchron nitroglycerin, as compared to 0.8 mg nitroglycerin administered sublingually, the mean pulmonary artery pressure values during exercise are significantly ($p < 0.05$) reduced (fig. 1). Figure 1 and table III clearly demonstrate that the effect of 0.8 mg nitroglycerin administered sublingually has subsided 180 min after application, resulting in the same mean pulmonary artery pressure during exercise as the premedication, i.e., in contrast to controlled-release nitroglycerin, no effect could be demonstrated for sublingually administered nitroglycerin at this point of time.

180 min after buccal application of 2.5 mg Synchron nitroglycerin, the absolute values for mean pulmonary artery pressure do not show statistically significant differences to those after 0.8 mg nitroglycerin sublingually

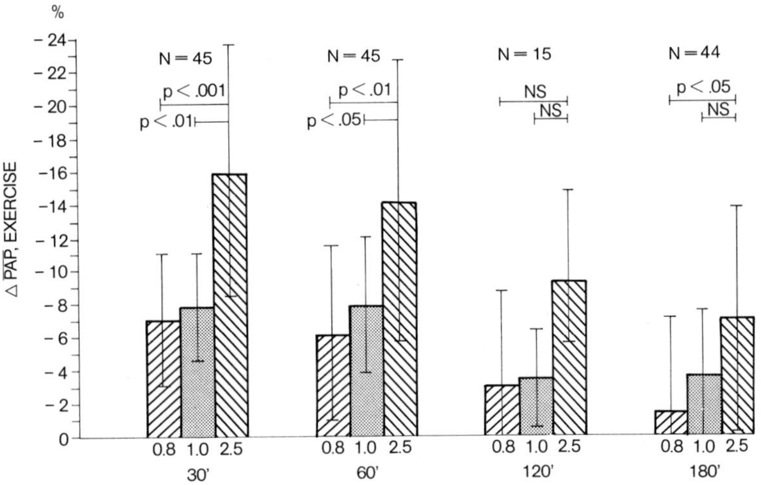

Fig. 6. Percent reduction of mean pulmonary artery pressure ($\overline{PAP}$, mm Hg) during exercise after application of 0.8, 1.0, or 2.5 mg nitroglycerin (mean ± SD).

because of high variation, whereas, compared to baseline values, the difference in reduction of mean pulmonary artery pressure is still ($p < 0.05$) statistically significant (fig. 6). We can also demonstrate that the effect of 0.8 mg nitroglycerin sublingually and 1.0 mg Synchron nitroglycerin buccally is similar after 30 min, despite different premedication pressure values, and that the effect of 1.0 mg Synchron nitroglycerin buccally persistes longer than that of 0.8 mg nitroglycerin sublingually. The total number of 45 patients was reduced by 1 during exercise at 180 min (fig. 6) since 1 patient from the group which received nitroglycerin sublingually was not in a position to exercise at his individual preselected work load, and exercise testing had to be terminated because of massive anginal symptoms and a pronounced ST segment depression.

Side-Effects, ECG Changes

During our study, the incidence of abnormal ECG changes, shown as ST segment depressions, did not differ significantly among the three test groups. 30 and 60 min after medication, ECG changes, classified as severe before medication, could no longer be established; 180 min after application the frequency of ECG changes slightly reincreased in the three groups. The incidence of anginal symptoms and dyspnea during exercise did not differ significantly in the three test groups.

After sublingual application of 0.8 mg nitroglycerin, 1 patient complained of mild headaches 30 min after application and another one 30 and 60 min after buccal administration of 2.5 mg Synchron nitroglycerin. In the same group 1 patient felt a dryness in the mouth 30 min after application.

Discussion

Nitroglycerin effects a reduction in pre- and afterload resulting in a diminished cardiac work load. A reliable parameter for the determination of a reduction in preload is the pulmonary artery pressure at rest and during exercise [1, 4, 5]. Since during exercise the mean pulmonary artery pressure shows a higher correlation to left ventricular end-diastolic pressure than the diastolic pulmonary pressure [2], we predominantly used the changes in mean pulmonary artery pressure for the evaluation of potency and duration of action of the various delivery and dosage forms of nitroglycerin. Buccally administered Synchron nitroglycerin and nitroglycerin sublingually did not differ significantly in their effect on resting and exercise heart rate and resting cardiac output. There is also only a mild effect on mean pulmonary artery pressure at rest with a significant difference only between 2.5 mg buccally administered Synchron nitroglycerin and 0.8 mg sublingually administered nitroglycerin 60 min after application when the maximum action of nitroglycerin sublingually is over. The study of the acute action of sublingually (0.8 mg) and buccally administered nitroglycerin (2.5 mg) under steady state condition shows their effect to be comparable, and during the subsequent resting phase the reduction in mean pulmonary artery pressure is also similar. 1.0 mg buccally administered Synchron nitroglycerin, however, doses not seem to have the same pronounced acute effect with a flatter curve under steady state as well as during the resting period compared to sublingually administered nitroglycerin, though the difference is not statistically significant (fig. 3, 4).

The mean pulmonary artery pressure values show a marked loss in action for nitroglycerin sublingually as early as 15 min after application. These results confirm those of other authors demonstrating the maximum of action after 10–15 min by determination of pulmonary artery pressure [3]. By contrast, after buccal application of 2.5 mg nitroglycerin – the same tendency after the 1.0-mg dose – there is a continuous reduction in mean pulmonary artery pressure at rest during the first 30 min to a maximum at 60 min; thus, we might assume a maximum of action between 30–60 min for this delivery form (fig. 1, 5, 6).

Compared with mean pulmonary artery pressure results, the analysis of nitroglycerin effects on systolic and diastolic pulmonary artery pressures among the three test drugs and the various work load did not add any further decisive aspects (table IV, V). 180 min after buccal application of 2.5 mg Synchron nitroglycerin, we found a statistically significant effect on systolic pulmonary artery pressure compared to 0.8 mg sublingually administered nitroglycerin (table III), demonstrating the longer duration of action after 2.5 mg Synchron nitroglycerin buccally in the same way as the percentage reduction of mean pulmonary artery pressure during exercise did (fig. 6), whereas the effects of 0.8 mg nitroglycerin sublingually and 1.0 mg Synchron nitroglycerin buccally show only minor differences. While the acute action of 1.0 mg buccally administered nitroglycerin is lower than that of nitroglycerin sublingually the duration of action is somewhat – but not significantly – longer with a maximum of action after 30–60 min determined by the reduction in mean pulmonary artery pressure (table III, fig. 1, 6). At 120 min, 2.5 mg Synchron nitroglycerin buccally has a pronounced effect on mean pulmonary artery pressure during exercise (fig. 1) whereas that of the 1.0-mg dose is only minor (fig. 1). Thus, we can state that the spectrum of activity of 0.8 mg nitroglycerin sublingually and 1.0 mg Synchron nitroglycerin buccally is similar, with nitroglycerin administered sublingually having a more pronounced acute effect and 1.0 mg nitroglycerin buccally a somewhat longer duration of action. After 2.5 mg Synchron nitroglycerin buccally, a statistically significant effect on mean pulmonary artery pressure and thus on the left ventricular end-diastolic pressure can be demonstrated as late as 180 min after medication in contrast to the effect of nitroglycerin administered sublingually. Its acute effect under steady state conditions and during the resting phase can be compared with nitroglycerin sublingually in its rapid onset of action and degree of reduction in pulmonary artery pressure. But nitroglycerin administered sublingually has its maximum of action 15 min after application whereas 2.5 mg Synchron nitroglycerin buccally only after 30–60 min, thus showing a statistically significant difference to sublingual nitroglycerin after 20 min and persisting up to 60 min after application. Compared to the 1.0-mg dose, the effect of 2.5 mg Synchron nitroglycerin buccally is more pronounced (table III, fig. 6); both dosage forms, however, have the same maximum of action in time. In interpreting the action at 180 min, the prolonged resting period has to be taken into account. The three test groups did not differ significantly in side-effects, ST segment changes, frequency of anginal attacks, and dyspnea.

Summarizing, we can state that 1.0 mg Synchron nitroglycerin administered buccally has a later onset of action and lower potency in acute therapy than 0.8 mg nitroglycerin sublingually. After 30 and 60 min, however, the effect on mean pulmonary artery pressure at rest and during exercise is somewhat more pronounced than that of nitroglycerin sublingually but is not significant. The maximum of action after 0.8 mg nitroglycerin administered sublingually is about 15 min after application, at 3 h no effect on mean pulmonary artery pressure can be demonstrated. After 2.5 mg Synchron nitroglycerin administered buccally, the onset of action is as rapid and the potency as high as after 0.8 mg nitroglycerin administered sublingually, but the duration of action persists – with a maximum of action after 30–60 min – over a longer period of time, and at 180 min effects can still be demonstrated. 2.5 mg Synchron nitroglycerin buccally has a faster and more potent effect than the 1.0-mg dose.

Synchron nitroglycerin administered buccally as 2.5-mg dosage form can be recommended as antianginal drug with a rapid onset and a long duration of action and, moreover, in comparison with other nitroglycerin formulations provides the advantage of therapeutic self-control by the patient.

References

1 Bollinger, A.; Fromm, U.; Brunner, H.H.; Mahler, F.; Casty, M.; Anliker, M.; Siegenthaler, W.: Die Wirkung von Isosorbiddinitrat (ISDN) auf den peripheren Kreislauf; in Rudolph, Siegenthaler, Nitrate, pp. 54–61 (Urban & Schwarzenberg, München 1976).

2 Bonzel, T.; Schmidt, H.; Sigwart, U.; Mertens, H.M.; Gleichmann, U.: Pulmonalarteriendrücke und linksventrikulärer enddiastolischer Druck in Ruhe und unter dynamischer Belastung. Z. Kardiol. *65:* 1088–1108 (1976).

3 Bussmann, W.-D.: Hämodynamik und Grösse des Myokardinfarktes bei Anwendung von Nitroglyzerin. 2. Hamburger Nitroglyzerin-Symposium 1979, pp. 125–133 (Pharmazeutische Verlagsgesellschaft, München 1980).

4 Karsch, K.R.; Rentrop, P.; Neuhaus, K.L.; Bornikoel, K.; Kreuzer, H.: Hämodynamik des rechten Ventrikels vor und nach Nitroglyzerin bei Patienten mit koronarer Herzkrankheit; in Rudolph, Schrey, Nitrate, vol. 2, pp. 193–198 (Urban & Schwarzenberg, München 1980).

5 Stauch, M.: Hämodynamik unter Nitraten im kleinen Kreislauf; in Rudolph, Siegenthaler, Nitrate, pp. 75–79 (Urban & Schwarzenberg, München 1976).

H. Ohlmeier, MD, Gollwitzer-Meier-Institut, Klinik für Herz- und Kreislauferkrankungen, Herforder Strasse 43, D-4970 Bad Oeynhausen (FRG)

Adv. Pharmacother., vol. 1, pp. 116–122 (Karger, Basel 1982)

Changes in Left Ventricular Hemodynamics under Buccal Synchron Nitroglycerin

A Noninvasive Study Using Systolic Time Intervals

H.M. Mertens, H. Ohlmeier, H. Mannebach, U. Gleichmann

Staatliches Gollwitzer-Meier-Institut, Klinik für Herz- und Kreislauferkrankungen (Prof. Dr. *U. Gleichmann*), Bad Oeynhausen, FRG

Introduction

Systolic time intervals (STI) are of great importance in the noninvasive evaluation of left ventricular function. Several investigators, particularly *Weissler* et al. [1], have shown a high correlation between hemodynamic parameters and STI [1, 2].

STI have proved to be a valuable method in clarifying pharmacologic questions [3, 5]. Results of nitrate compound action on STI have been published among others by *Simon* et al. [6], *Harris* et al. [7] and *Sawayama* et al. [8].

The aim of our study was the documentation of intensity and duration of action of buccal Synchron nitroglycerin in comparison to sublingual nitroglycerin by determination of STI.

Material and Methods

In a randomized study 32 patients (30 men, 2 women, mean age 41.2 years) with coronary heart disease, documented by coronary arteriography, and left ventricular dysfunction, documented with a floating catheter, received 0.8 mg sublingual nitroglycerin (11 patients) or buccal Synchron nitroglycerin at a dosage of 1.0 mg (11 patients) or 2.5 mg (10 patients). The groups were homogeneous in age and severity of coronary heart disease or left ventricular dysfunction. Before the study, any administration of negative or positive inotropic drugs was discontinued.

Identical times of the day were chosen for all examinations. STI were determined in a supine position before and 30, 60 and 180 min after drug administration. Simultaneous recording of electrocardiogram, phonocardiogram and indirect carotid arterial pulse curve (paper speed 100 mm/s) were used to measure the following parameters: heart rate, electromechanical systole QS_2 (the period from the onset of the QRS complex to the first high-frequency deflection of the second heart sound), left ventricular ejection time LVET (begins with the upstroke of the carotid arterial pulse and ends with the incisura), preejection period PEP (difference between QS_2 and LVET), as well as the preejection and ejection time ratio PEP/LVET. The mean value from five consecutive heart cycles was calculated [9]. The t-test was used for statistic analysis and significance assumed on the 5% level.

Results

Changes in heart rate and STI after administration of sublingual nitroglycerin caps and of buccal Synchron nitroglycerin tablets are summarized in table I and figure 1.

Heart Rate. There are no specific significant changes in heart rate during the time of application or between different dosage forms of nitroglycerin. 30 min after buccal administration of 2.5 mg Synchron nitroglycerin, a pronounced rise in heart rate was observed but a significant change against baseline values could not be demonstrated statistically.

QS_2. The electromechanical systole does not show any specific, significant changes against baseline values, between dosage forms or in relation to

Table I. Mean values and standard deviation of heart rate (HR, beats per minute), preejection period (PEP, milliseconds), ejection time (LVET, milliseconds) and the ratio of preejection period and ejection time (PEP/LVET) before and after (30, 60 and 180 min) application of 0.8 mg sublingual nitroglycerin or 1.0 or 2.5 mg buccal Synchron nitroglycerin

Minutes after application	Buccal 1.0 mg (n=11)	Buccal 2.5 mg (n=10)	Sublingual 0.8 mg (n=11)	Buccal 1.0 mg (n=11)	Buccal 2.5 mg (n=10)	Sublingual 0.8 mg (n=11)
	HR			*PEP*		
0	73±12	71±11	75±11	108± 7	107±13	103±10
30	76±14	79±14	73±12	116± 8	119±12	116± 7
60	74±14	75±15	73±12	122± 7	123±12	112±11
180	70±13	67± 9	68±12	121± 9	118±15	111±13
	LVET			*PEP/LVET*		
0	281±22	280±27	288±28	387±37	364±52	355±30
30	265±18	246±27	270±24	440±41	486±61	431±44
60	264±22	248±30	275±25	464±54	505±64	409±51
180	276±26	275±27	292±27	442±65	430±59	382±55

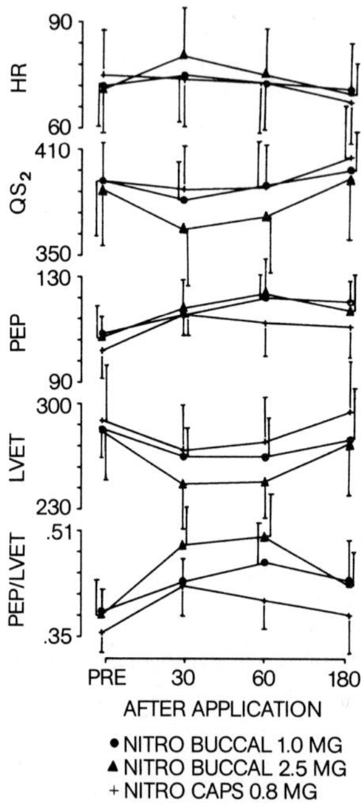

Fig. 1. Mean value and standard deviation of heart rate (HR, beats/min), electromechanical systole (QS_2, msec), preejection period (PEP, msec), ejection time (LVET, msec) and the ratio of preejection period and ejection time (PEP/LVET) before and after application of 0.8 mg sublingual nitroglycerin or 1.0 mg or 2.5 mg buccal Synchron nitroglycerin.

time. We shall abstain from any further discussion of these findings because of the – in our eyes – minor hemodynamic significance of these parameters.

PEP. 30, 60 and 180 min after administration of nitroglycerin the preejection period lengthens in all three groups. 30 min after sublingual administration of 0.8 mg nitroglycerin this prolongation is statistically significant ($p \leq 0.01$).

60 and 180 min after 1 mg buccal Synchron nitroglycerin application PEP is significantly lengthened ($p < 0.001$ or $p \leq 0.01$).

The administration of 2.5 mg buccal Synchron nitroglycerin effects a significant prolongation of PEP after 30 and 60 min ($p \leq 0.05$ or $p \leq 0.01$).

In the predrug phase PEP did not show any significant differences between the drug groups. This was still true 30 min after administration of the test drug. 60 min after application of 1.0 and 2.5 mg buccal Synchron nitroglycerin the prolongation of PEP is significantly greater than that after 0.8 mg sublingual nitroglycerin ($p \leq 0.05$). There is no significant difference between 1.0 and 2.5 mg buccal Synchron nitroglycerin tablets. 180 min after application, significant differences between the drug groups can no longer be detected.

LVET. There were no significant left ventricular ejection time changes in relation to time and between the two drug groups of 0.8 mg sublingual nitroglycerin and 1.0 mg buccal Synchron nitroglycerin. 30 and 60 min after application of 2.5 mg buccal Synchron nitroglycerin LVET is significantly shortened ($p \leq 0.05$) and after 180 min significantly re-increased towards the baseline value ($p \leq 0.05$). There were no detectable differences in action between 1.0 mg and 2.5 mg buccal Synchron nitroglycerin but the diminishment of LVET after 30 and 60 min was significantly greater with 2.5 mg buccal Synchron nitroglycerin than with 0.8 mg sublingual nitroglycerin ($p \leq 0.05$).

PEP/LVET. No significant differences exist between the drug groups' baseline values of PEP/LVET ratio, and in all three dosage forms a significant ratio increase is detected after 30 and 60 min. After sublingual administration of 0.8 mg nitroglycerin, PEP/LVET lengthens from 355 to 431 or 409 ($p \leq 0.001$ or $p \leq 0.01$).

2.5 mg buccal Synchron nitroglycerin effects the PEP/LVET prolongation by an increase from 364 to 486 or 505 after 30 to 60 min ($p \leq 0.001$ and $p \leq 0.001$).

After application of 1.0 mg buccal Synchron nitroglycerin the PEP/LVET ratio increases from 387 to 440 ($p \leq 0.05$) or 464 ($p \leq 0.01$).

30 min after medication, 2.5 mg buccal Synchron nitroglycerin leads to a significantly greater increase in the PEP/LVET ratio than 0.8 mg sublingual nitroglycerin ($p \leq 0.05$). At this time a quantitative difference of action between 1.0 and 2.5 mg buccal Synchron nitroglycerin and between 0.8 mg sublingual nitroglycerin and 1.0 mg buccal Synchron nitroglycerin cannot be demonstrated statistically.

60 min after administration of 1.0-mg as well as 2.5-mg buccal Synchron nitroglycerin tablets, the prolongation of PEP/LVET is significantly greater than after sublingual application of 0.8-mg nitroglycerin caps ($p \leq 0.01$ or $p \leq 0.05$). A difference of action between 1.0 and 2.5 mg buccal Synchron nitroglycerin cannot be demonstrated statistically at this interval, either.

Discussion

In our investigation the heart rate at rest is not significantly affected by buccal Synchron nitroglycerin or sublingual nitroglycerin. The systolic time intervals, however, clearly show typical changes: prolongation of the preejection period PEP and shortening of ejection time LVET. Since prolongation of the preejection period PEP is more pronounced than shortening of LVET, a marked increase in the PEP/LVET ratio results. Table II shows a selection of parameters for left ventricular function and peripheral circulation correlating positively or negatively with the STI.

The prolongation of PEP, the shortening of LVET and the resulting increase in the PEP/LVET ratio under nitroglycerin should not be misinterpreted as an increasing congestive heart failure of the left ventricle. The PEP increase under nitroglycerin results from a pronounced reduction in the pre-

Table II. Relation between systolic time intervals and changes in left ventricular hemodynamics, changes in peripheral circulation parameters and pharmacologic intervention

Increase	Decrease
PEP	
LVEDP ↑	LVEDP ↓
negative-inotropic drugs	positive inotropic drugs
contractility ↓	contractility ↑
blood pressure (diastolic) ↑	blood pressure (diastolic) ↓
afterload ↑	afterload ↓
preload ↓	preload ↑
LVET	
LVEDP ↓	LVEDP ↑
blood pressure (systolic) ↑	blood pressure (systolic) ↓
positive inotropic drugs	negative and positive inotropic drugs
afterload ↑	afterload ↓
stroke volume ↑	stroke volume ↓
preload ↑	preload ↓
PEP/LVET	
negative inotropic drugs	positive inotropic drugs
contractility ↓	contractility ↑
LVEDP ↑	LVEDP ↓
venous pooling ↑	venous pooling ↓
blood pressure ↑	blood pressure ↓
ejection fraction ↓	ejection fraction ↑

load and the shortening of LVET from a decrease in systolic blood pressure and a reduction of the pre- and afterload. The well-known mechanisms of venous pooling lead to a considerably reduced venous return and thus to a marked increase in the PEP/LVET ratio [6, 10].

Analyzing the data in respect of duration of action shows that the greatest differences of STI from baseline values are observed 30 min after sublingual administration of 0.8 mg nitroglycerin. Thereafter and up to a period of 180 min the data approximate baseline values.

After administering 1.0 or 2.5 mg buccal Synchron nitroglycerin, the greatest differences to basline values were registered as late as 60 min after application and after 180 min a trend towards baseline values was observed.

Consequently, after sublingual administration of 0.8 mg nitroglycerin, maximum action related to STI is reached or even exceeded after 30 min, whereas that of buccal Synchron nitroglycerin tablets is reached as late as 60 min after application, irrespective of dosage form. The interpretation of the 180-min data is difficult. No detectable effects can be demonstrated after sublingual application of 0.8 mg nitroglycerin. After application of 1.0 mg or 2.5 mg buccal Synchron nitroglycerin, the 180-min data clearly differ from baseline values (but are not statistically significant). These values, however, are influenced by the effect of a 3-hour resting period as indicated by the heart rate, clearly below baseline values in all three study groups after 180 min. To sum up, a duration of action up to 60 min can be demonstrated for 1.0- and 2.5-mg buccal Synchron nitroglycerin tablets and a duration of action up to 180 min is probable.

Quantitative differences in action between sublingual nitroglycerin caps and buccal Synchron nitroglycerin tablets could not be demonstrated as maximum action of sublingual nitroglycerin is already exceeded after 30 min whereas that of buccal Synchron nitroglycerin is only reached after 60 min.

The 2.5-mg tablet of buccal Synchron nitroglycerin effects greater changes in all parameters of STI against the baseline values than the 1.0 mg dose. These differences, however, are not statistically significant because of the interindividual variation.

References

1 Weissler, A.M.; Harris, W.S.; Schoenfeld, C.D.: Bedside technics for the evaluation of ventricular function in man. Am. J. Cardiol. *23:* 577 (1969).

2 Weissler, A.M.: Systolic time intervals. New Engl. J. Med. *296:* 321 (1977).

3 Buch, H.; Egeblad, H.; Hansen, P.B.; Kjaergard, H.; Waldorff, S.; Steiness, E.: Correlation

between changes in systolic time intervals and left ventricular end-diastolic diameter after preload reduction. Br. Heart J. *44:* 668–671 (1980).

4 Kuhn, H.; Jaeschke, M.; Breithardt, G.; Loogen, F.: Zur kardialen Wirkung von Glucagon. Untersuchungen bei Patienten mit chronischer Herzinsuffizienz. Z. Kardiol. *57:* 256 (1978).

5 Breithardt, G.; Jochum, E.; Kuhn, H.; Seipel, L.: Die Wirkung verschiedener Antiarrhythmika auf die systolischen Zeitintervalle bei Normalpersonen. Z. Kardiol. *67:* 680 (1978).

6 Simon, H.; Schuppen, U.; Bähre, M.; Breuel, H.P.: Akutwirkung von Nitroverbindungen auf das Myokard bei koronarer Herzerkrankung. 2. Deutsches Nitroglyzerin Symp. 1979, p. 29 (Pharmazeut. Verlagsgesellschaft, München 1980).

7 Harris, W.S.; Aytan, N.; Pouget, J.M.: Effects of nitroglycerin on responses of the systolic time intervals to exercise. Circulation *47:* 499 (1973).

8 Sawayama, T.; Masakazu, O.; Marumoto, S.; Matsuura, T.; Niki, J.: Influence of amyl nitride inhalation on the systolic time intervals in normal subjects and in patients with ischemic heart disease. Circulation *40:* 327 (1969).

9 Mertens, H.M.; Mannebach, H.; Trieb, G.; Gleichmann, U.: Influence of heart rate on systolic time intervals: effects of atrial pacing versus dynamic exercise. Clin. Cardiol. *4:* 22 (1981).

10 Kuhn, H.; Loogen, F.: Die Bestimmung der systolischen Zeitintervalle. Dt. med. Wschr. *105:* 214–218 (1980).

H.M. Mertens, MD, Staatliches Gollwitzer-Meier-Institut, Klinik für Herz- und Kreislauferkrankungen, Herforder Strasse 43, D-4970 Bad Oeynhausen (FRG)

Discussion

Chairmen: *U. Gleichmann* and *N. Reichek*

Bussmann: What are your experiences with 5.0 mg buccal nitroglycerin?

Ohlmeier: We only tested it in a pre-phase when we wanted to see what effects might be expected. I think with one patient without measuring pulmonary artery mean pressure we had fatigue and he had to lie down. With another man we had a really impressive down-sloping of pulmonary artery mean pressure.

Adv. Pharmacother., vol. 1, pp. 123–136 (Karger, Basel 1982)

Cold-Induced Angina pectoris

Acute Prophylaxis and Long-Term Protection by Controlled-Release Buccal Nitroglycerin[1]

Gerold Prager[a], *Wolfgang Wagner*[b]

[a] Regensburg, [b] Dortmund, FRG

Introduction

During cold exposure, central thermic homeostasis is kept constant due to certain protective mechanisms triggered off by baroreceptors [1–3]. The first protective response is a peripheral vasoconstriction leading to centralization of blood flow and to an increase in blood pressure. The second mechanism is an enhanced metabolism bringing about higher oxygen consumption and a higher cardiac output. Both mechanisms produce an abrupt increase in cardiac work load, and patients with coronary heart disease suffer from a sudden drop in work capacity and increased angina pectoris symptoms.

Some authors described the possibility of coronary vasospasms producing cold-induced angina pectoris [4–7]. Numerous studies on hemodynamic parameters during cold exposure have already been performed on healthy subjects [8–16] and on patients with cold-induced angina pectoris [4–7, 17–24]. All these investigations were carried out in laboratories under constant and reproducible conditions. Until now there has been no discussion on the effect of cold exposure in patients with ischemic heart disease produced in their normal home or work environment. There are also no reports on therapeutic management of cold-induced angina pectoris.

This study was designed to examine the reactions of patients with ischemic heart disease during cold exposure and the possibility of statistically significant results to be achieved by investigating the effect of drugs on cold-

[1] We would like to thank Miss *Kraupner* for her kind and helpful assistance while taking care of the patients.

induced angina pectoris. The efficacy of buccally administered Synchron nitroglycerin in respect of acute prophylactic and long-term protection was studied using a long-term ECG and clinical data.

Patients and Methods

Patients

The study comprised 33 patients ranging in age from 47 to 73 years with a mean age of 62 years. 33% of the patients were female and 67% male. In all patients, coronary heart disease was documented by a careful history and linear ST segment depression of ≧ 0.15 mV during exercise testing. Moreover, coronary angiograms were taken for most of them. During exercise ischemic reactions occurred at a work load of 50–125 W.

Prior to the study the patients suffered from cold-induced angina between 1 and 207 months, an average of 34 months. In most cases clinical manifestation of a coronary heart disease coincided with primary manifestation of cold-induced angina pectoris.

Besides previous myocardial infarction and severe acute or chronic systemic disorders, the main criterion for exclusion from the study was the occurrence of spontaneous angina pectoris attacks.

Careful compliance and cooperation on the part of the patients was a precondition for a successful outcome of this study. All patients were extensively informed about purpose, type and extent of the study, and written consent was obtained.

Methods

Study Design. Using a double-blind, crossover protocol, buccally administered Synchron nitroglycerin (1.0 mg) and placebo were compared on 2 consecutive days under normal conditions. Placebo and the active test drug were applied in a randomized sequence on different days. The acute prophylactic effect was studied by exposing patients to cold directly after their breakfast in the morning and after having administered the test substance. Long-term protection was examined by another two cold exposures at approximately 60-min intervals (fig. 1).

Test Procedures and Measurements. At 2 p.m. on the day prior to the study, a long-term ECG was performed, and the test substance I, two thermometers, and a booklet were handed over. The two thermometers were mounted in the patients' home and outdoors. During cold exposure indoor and outdoor temperatures were recorded.

The test substance was applied buccally after a normal breakfast. The patient was instructed to behave as usual after 5 min, i.e., walk to the garage, go for a walk with the dog, or take up other domestic jobs.

During the second and third exposure the patients were instructed to carry on in the same way. The time of cold exposure was recorded in the patients' protocol as well as the duration of the anginal episode.

The marker of the long-term ECG recorder was used to characterize the following events: (1) time of test substance application; (2) onset of anginal attack, and (3) the end of the anginal attack (fig. 2).

In the afternoon the patient returned for exchange of the long-term ECG cassette. The electrodes were reset to avoid skin irritation, and the patients' records were discussed with him.

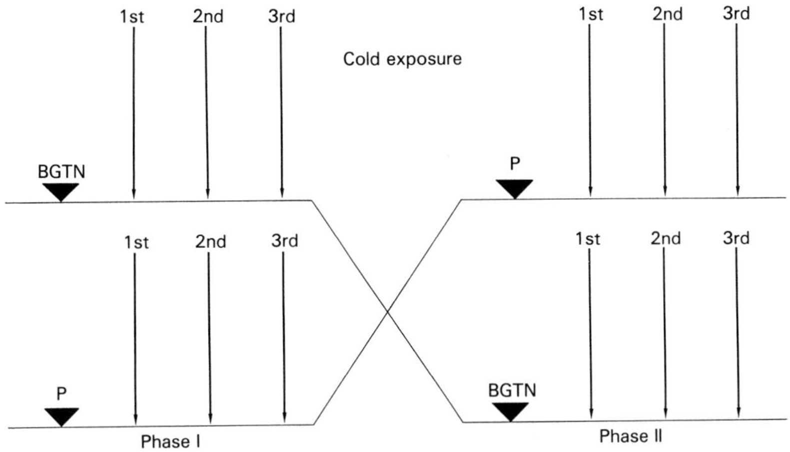

Fig. 1. Study design. Buccally administered Synchron nitroglycerin (BGTN; 1 mg); placebo as a buccal tablet (P).

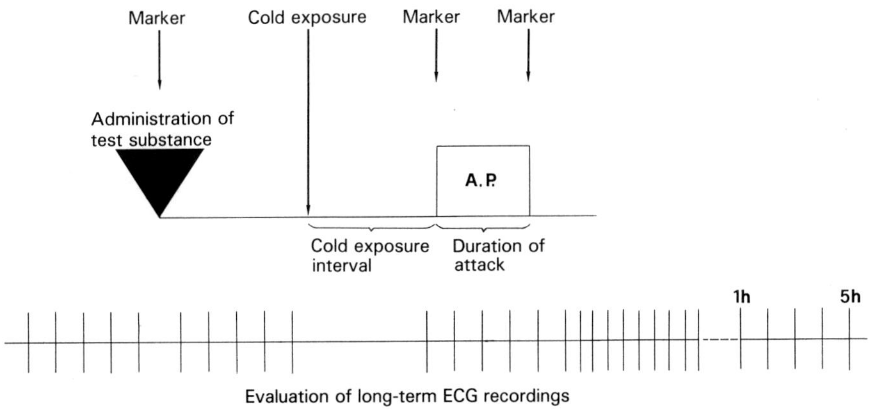

Fig. 2. Measurements during the first exposure to cold.

Thereafter he received test substance II. The second test phase did not differ from the first one with the patient returning the next afternoon for removal of the long-term ECG recorder.

Long-term ECG analysis was performed with an Oxford M 2A-HL 8 analysis system using a medilog 2 recorder. Time marking was done by the patient pressing a push button. This is shown as a spike and easily located in the long-term ECG.

ST segment displacement and heart rate were recorded in a histogram over 24 h – 30 mm corresponding to 1 h – to indicate tendencies. The system does not include ST segment shifts recorded via a fixed point in the ST segment to a fixed reference point at the QRS complex; form changes cannot be shown. An automatic analysis of pathological ST segment depressions is thus

Table I. Incidence of cold exposures at different outdoor temperatures

Outdoor temperature, °C	Cold exposures	
	n	%
≤–5	25	14.2
–4.9–0	58	33.0
0.1–5	52	29.5
> 5	41	23.3
Total	176	100.0

Table II. Incidence of test substances and cold exposures at different outdoor temperatures

Outdoor temperature, °C	Test substances		Total number of cold exposures	
	active drug	placebo	n	%
≤ 0	41	42	83	47.2
> 0	45	48	93	52.8
Total	86	90	176	100.0

Table III. Incidence of test substances and cold exposures at different degrees of severity of the coronary artery disease, measured by exercise tolerance

Exercise tolerance	Test substances		Total number of cold exposures	
	active drug	placebo	n	%
> 75	13	12	25	14.5
≤ 75	71	76	147	85.5
Total	84	88	172	100.0

not possible since the system cannot discriminate between ascending and linear or descending ST depression. Therefore, heart rate and ST segment depression were measured 'manually' using ECG strips recorded at planned protocol intervals and at the times marked by the patient. The electrodes were positioned in such a way that the recorded QRS complex resembled that of lead V 5 and another that of lead V 1. Directly before and after application of the test substance, an ECG was written 5 times and then at intervals of 1–5 h. Further ECG recordings were made at the time of cold exposure and in individual cases between 1 and 5 times during the anginal episode.

Except with long-acting nitrates any therapy with beta-blocking agents and calcium antagonists was continued. To manage the anginal attack the patient stood still or applied a sublingual nitroglycerin capsule.

The following variables were evaluated: (1) long-term ECG: ST segment depression and heart rate and (2) clinical data: indoor and outdoor temperatures, episode of angina pectoris, interval up to the anginal attack (cold exposure interval), and the duration of the anginal attack.

Indoor and Outdoor Temperature. The patients measured an indoor temperature of 19–22 °C. The mean temperature of cold exposure was −1 °C. The intra- and interindividual variations were considerable with maximum temperatures between −13 and +10 °C. Table I shows the incidence using a four-grade classification. *Freedberg* et al. [4] and *Wayne and Graybiel* [17] also described 'responses to cold' at exposure temperatures of +6 to +13 °C.

Statistical Analysis. The inconsistency of study conditions prevented a one-way analogous evaluation by an analysis of variance for our crossover design. Further statistical methods had to be used, among them were: (1) one-way analysis of variance; (2) t test for independent samples; (3) χ^2-test, and (4) combination of fourfold tables.

A four-grade classification was used to study the correlation between temperature at the time of cold exposure and severity of coronary heart disease after exercise stress testing. But due to the low frequency in subgroups and the resulting inconsistent trends, we decided in favor of a more general stratification with two grades and the following incidence to evaluate the variables 'temperature' (table II) and 'severity' (table III).

Results and Discussion

Casuistical and statistical analyses were used for the evaluation of clinical and electrocardiographic data.

Casuistic Analysis

Two major findings were of interest: (1) An ST segment elevation did not occur in any patient at any point of time, neither immediately after cold exposure nor during or after anginal attacks. This is of significance and means that, in our study, coronary artery spasm did not seem to play an important role in initiating cold-induced angina pectoris. (2) A few cases of dysrhythmias occurred, some of a malignant nature, in 1 case with ventricular flutter

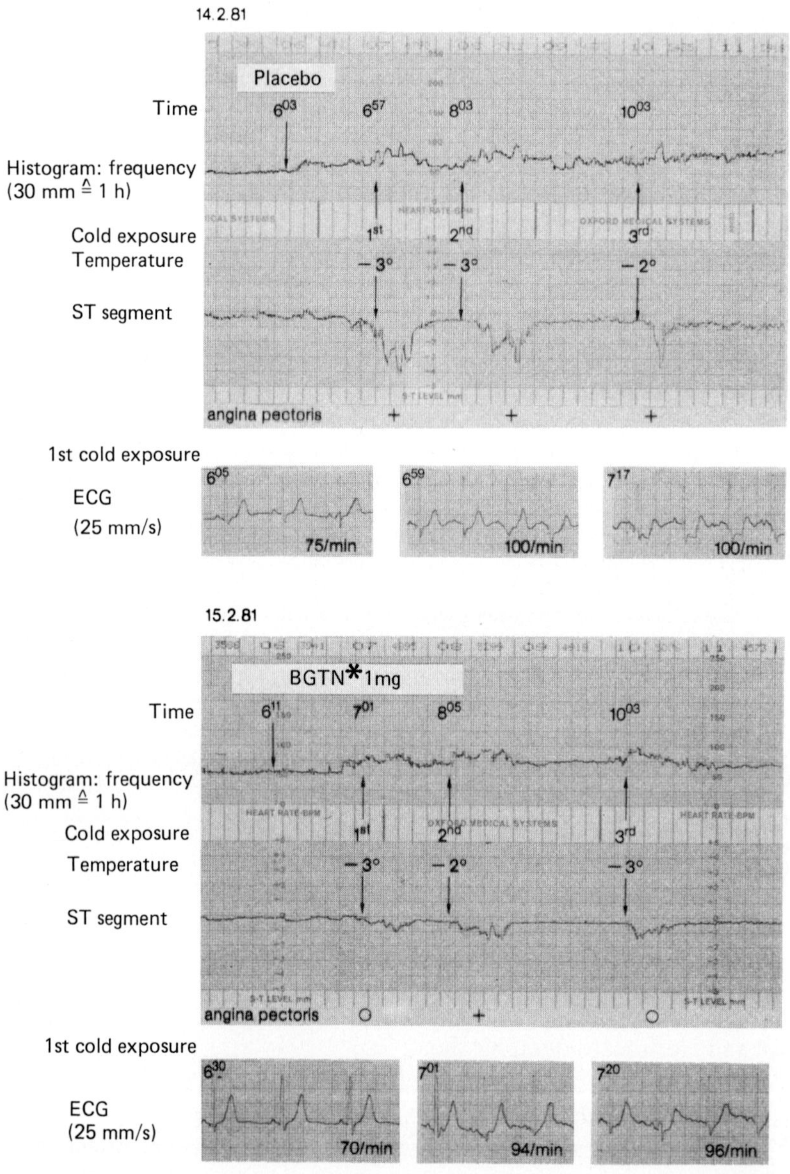

Fig. 3. Acute prophylactic and protracted effect of controlled-release buccal Synchron nitroglycerin (1 mg) vs. placebo in a 62-year-old patient with stable coronary heart disease during cold exposure under the same conditions of examination, represented by means of long-term ECG.

paroxysm. We did not examine any arrhythmias after exposure to cold because previous research work described them to be of no significance [18].

Case 1 (fig. 3) demonstrates the phenomenology of cold exposure and the protection by buccally administered nitroglycerin. In a 62-year-old patient with stable coronary heart disease of grade II, a definite increase in heart rate from 75 to 100 beats/min occurred when changing from room temperature of +22 °C to an outdoor temperature of −3 °C. After some time of cold exposure the anginal attack was not accompanied by any further relevant increase in heart rate. The maximum ST segment depression of 0.4 mV was not observed at the onset of the anginal episode but in the second third of it. The attack was relieved by resting, i.e., standing still. The second and third cold exposure at the same temperature produced identical responses.

On the next day, Synchron nitroglycerin was administered buccally under virtually the same conditions – application of the test substance and cold exposure at the same time and outdoor temperature again −3 °C. However, after application of the test agent the patient had no anginal attack during the first and third cold exposure. During the second cold exposure an anginal attack occurred, but the ST segment depression was considerably lower, being only 0.1 mV.

The acute prophylactic and astonishingly sustained duration of action of buccally administered nitroglycerin is shown in the fact that the drug was administered almost 1 h before cold exposure and its protective effect persisted over 4 h up to the third cold exposure. These very encouraging results seem to justify the design and implementation of this research study.

Case 2, a 59-year-old man, illustrates special problems inherent in a study under normal everyday conditions: table IV shows the cold exposure interval, the duration of anginal attack, and the maximum ST segment depression. After application of nitroglycerin the exposure interval was considerably prolonged, the duration of attack shortened, and ST segment depression considerably improved. There are, however, a few difficulties in relating these positive effects directly and exclusively to the action of buccally administered Synchron nitroglycerin. The test temperature during the first and second cold exposure was up to 9 °C higher after application of the active test agent.

Statistical Analysis

Heart Rate. In the predrug phase cold exposure immediately produced an increase in heart rate and led to an anginal attack with continually increas-

Table IV. Problems of interpreting the therapeutic effect in a 59-year-old patient at different degrees of temperature in both test phases: limits of testing under normal everyday conditions

	Cold exposure		
	1st	2nd	3rd
Placebo (February 20, 1981)			
Cold exposure interval, min	3	4	6
Duration of attack, min	3	3	5
Maximum ST depression during attack, mV	0.7	0.6	0.7
Temperature at the time of cold exposure, °C	–4	–3	+3
Buccally applied nitroglycerin (1 mg; February 21, 1981)			
Cold exposure interval, min	9	8	13
Duration of attack, min	2	2	2
Maximum ST depression during attack, mV	0.4	0.2	0.5
Temperature at the time of cold exposure, °C	+5	+5	+4

Table V. Mean heart rate in relation to outdoor temperature and exercise tolerance under placebo (mean ± SD)

	Heart rate, beats/min
Outdoor temperature, °C	
≤ 0	105.0 ± 17.7
> 0	99.0 ± 17.4
Exercise tolerance, W	
> 75	93.2 ± 18.6
≤ 75	106.6 ± 21.0

Table VI. Maximum mean ST segment depression during anginal attack in relation to outdoor temperature and exercise tolerance under nitroglycerin (mean ± SD)

	ST segment depression, mV
Outdoor temperature, °C	
≤ 0	0.219 ± 0.177
> 0	0.167 ± 0.101
Exercise tolerance, W	
> 75	0.167 ± 0.166
≤ 75	0.200 ± 0.143

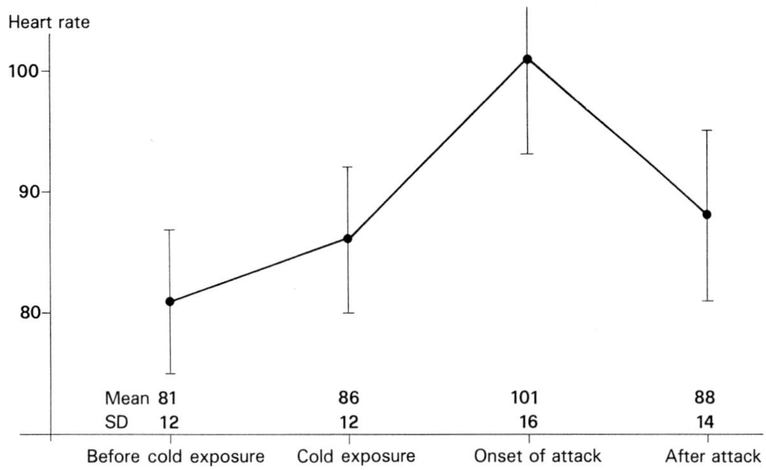

Fig. 4. Time course of heart rate during cold exposure and anginal attack after application of placebo.

ing heart rate. After the attack a pronounced decrease in heart rate was observed (fig. 4).

The heart rate after application of placebo and the active test substance did not differ significantly, but a correlation between temperature and severity of the coronary artery disease was clearly evident. The increase in heart rate correlated with reduced outdoor temperature and diminished exercise tolerance (table V).

ST Segment Displacement. Cold exposure after placebo is only rarely followed by ST segment depression. During an anginal attack, a maximum of 0.20 mV (mean value) and an absolute maximum of 0.7 mV were observed. An ST segment elevation was never observed during cold exposure. The maximal ST segment depression did not occur at onset, but during the second third of the attack. This was most pronounced in anginal attacks that were relieved by resting, i.e., standing still (see also histogram in figure 3).

ST segment displacement did not differ significantly in the placebo and test drug group. In the subgroups a clear correlation to temperature was observed with the maximal ST depression more pronounced at colder temperatures. A similar trend with correlation to the severity of coronary artery disease was only observed in the active test drug group (table VI).

Duration of Attack. After application of placebo, the mean duration of an anginal attack was 5.3 min with an absolute minimum value of 1 min and an absolute maximum of 22 min. There was no significant difference in duration of attack after application of placebo and nitroglycerin. The statistical analysis of subgroups did not show any correlation to temperature, but a good correlation to the severity of coronary heart disease, i.e., the attack duration increases with severity of coronary heart disease in the placebo and nitroglycerin groups (table VII).

Frequency of Anginal Attacks. During the control phase an angina pectoris attack is observed in 60% of the cases after cold exposure. Again, there is no statistically significant difference between the placebo and nitroglycerin group, and the same is true for the correlation to temperature. However, in relation to the severity of coronary heart disease a significant trend emerges showing a higher incidence of anginal attacks with higher severity after cold exposure.

After placebo the three-grade classification shows a 92% anginal frequency after exposure during exercise with a work load of $\leqq 50$ W and only 61% during exercise with > 75 W. After placebo the statistical difference in severity of coronary artery disease is $p = 0.043$.

Cold Exposure Interval. The cold exposure interval is defined as the time from the start of cold exposure to the onset of angina pectoris. The time interval represents the individual residual capacity of performance in patients with coronary artery disease. Based on a mean value of 8.9 min with high variation (minimum 2 min, maximum 34 min) in the predrug phase, a good correlation to temperature and severity of the disease becomes evident. The correlation of cold exposure interval and severity of coronary heart disease was statistically highly significant, being $p = 0.001$. The placebo data are shown in table VIII.

The correlation to exposure temperature shows a clear trend as well. Using the four-grade classification, the mean exposure interval is 6.6 min at below $-5\,^{\circ}$C, but 14 min at a temperature above $+5\,^{\circ}$C.

Therapeutic Effect on Cold Exposure Interval. As shown in figure 5a, on the left, the total group has a marked prolongation of cold exposure interval of an average of 3 min after buccal application of Synchron nitroglycerin. The therapeutic effect is thus statistically highly significant ($p = 0.001$).

In figure 5b not only an acute prophylactic effect during initial cold

Table VII. Mean duration of anginal attack in relation to exercise tolerance during administration of placebo (mean ± SD)

Exercise tolerance, W	Duration of attack, min
≤ 75	3.6 ± 1.8
> 75	5.0 ± 4.0

Table VIII. Mean cold exposure interval in relation to severity of the coronary artery disease under placebo (mean ± SD)

Exercise tolerance, W	Cold exposure, min
> 75	13.5 ± 8.3
≤ 75	8.0 ± 4.8

exposure can be demonstrated, but also a therapeutic long-term protection with a statistically significant prolongation of the exposure interval during the second and third cold exposure ($p = 0.001$). As can be seen from the annex to this study, the long-term protection persists on average over 3 h. Complementary to figure 5, table IX shows the cold exposure intervals for the patients who received first BGTN and then placebo. The analysis of variance shows a significant difference in favor of BGTN ($p = 0.0013$). The crossed-over group shows similar results based on a smaller number of cold exposures.

All test parameters showed a linear correlation to cold exposure temperatures and severity of coronary heart disease. Heart rate, maximal ST segment depression during the attack, duration of attack, and anginal frequency showed a more or less pronounced tendency. The correlation between cold exposure interval and severity of coronary artery disease was statistically highly significant. The linear characteristics of these parameters seem to demonstrate that cold exposure mainly presents an acute or chronic work load or stress for the heart, possibly triggered off by protective mechanisms. Coronary artery spasms, on the other hand, would be expected to lead to higher variation in parameters with wide scattering. Another argument against vasospastic genesis is the fact that no ST segment elevations were observed. Thus, we can state that in our patient population, selective in not including patients with spontaneous angina pectoris, vasospastic trigger mechanisms evidently did not play a role.

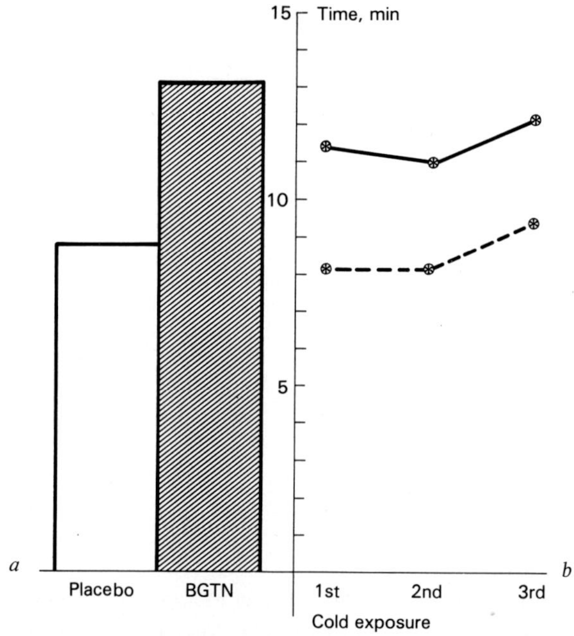

Fig. 5. *a* The total patient population shows a significant prolongation of the mean interval between onset of cold exposure and anginal attack (cold exposure interval) after buccal application of 1 mg Synchron nitroglycerin (BGTN; p=0.001). *b* Mean cold exposure intervals for individual cold exposures. Significant prolongation of each cold exposure interval after BGTN (p=0.001). —— = BGTN; – – – = placebo.

Table IX. Mean cold exposure intervals for the individual cold exposures under buccal Synchron nitroglycerin and placebo (mean ± SD)

Cold exposure	n	Mean ± SD
Nitroglycerin		
1st	12	11.4 ± 8.0
2nd	12	11.1 ± 5.5
3rd	11	12.3 ± 12.5
Placebo		
1st	16	8.2 ± 4.1
2nd	9	8.2 ± 4.1
3rd	9	9.4 ± 5.5
Intraindividual values		
Nitroglycerin	17	13.1 ± 10.0
Placebo	16	8.9 ± 4.1

The most sensitive parameter for demonstrating the drug effect under normal everyday conditions was the cold exposure interval. The cold exposure interval represents the residual capacity of performance of the patient. An increase in cold exposure interval means an increase in exercise tolerance. The therapeutic success of buccally administered Synchron nitroglycerin was statistically highly significant.

Conclusion

Summarizing, we can state that cold-induced angina pectoris is generated by protective reflex mechanisms leading to an abrupt decrease in cardiac performance due to an abrupt increase in cardiac work load.

In the present study there is no evidence of coronary artery spasm playing a role in patients with stable coronary heart disease. The clinical phenomena of 33 patients with stable angina pectoris were studied under everyday conditions using the long-term ECG technique and a double-blind crossover protocol. Included in the study was the evaluation of drug management for cold-induced angina pectoris.

Acute prophylaxis and long-term protection after application of buccally administered controlled-release nitroglycerin (1 mg) are demonstrated by casuistic examples and confirmed by statistics in comparison to placebo. After buccal application of Synchron nitroglycerin, a statistically highly significant prolongation of cold exposure interval can be observed which represents an increase in cardiac performance.

References

1 Ahnefeld, F.W.; Klingebiel, H.; Mehrkens, H.H.: Pathophysiologie und Therapie von Kälteschäden. Medsche Klin. *74:* 1833–1841 (1979).

2 Neureuther, G.; Flora, G.: Kälteschäden. Notfallmedizin *4:* 103–108 (1978).

3 Mehrkens, H.H.: Kälteschäden und thermische Läsionen. Z. Allgemeinmed. *57:* 209–221 (1981).

4 Freedberg, A.S.; Spiegl, E.D.; Riseman, J.E.F.: Effect of external heat and cold on patients with angina pectoris: evidence for the existence of a reflex factor. Am. Heart J. *27:* 611 (1944).

5 Mudge, G.H., Jr.; Grossman, W.; Mills, R.M.; Lesch, M.; Braunwald, E.: Reflex increase in coronary vascular resistance in patients with ischemic heart disease. New Engl. J. Med. *295:* 1333–1337.

6 Hattenhauer, M.; Neill, W.A.: The effect of cold air inhalation on angina pectoris and myocardial oxygen supply. Circulation *51:* 1053–1058 (1975).
7 Kober, G.; Wendt, T.; Schulz, W.; Kaltenbach, M.: Detection of coronary spasm by exposure to cold air and water. Int. Symp. on New Aspects of Unstable Angina, Hannover 1980.
8 Le Blanc, J.; Girard, B.; Dulac, S.; Côté, J.: The autonomic nervous system in cold adaption. J. appl. Physiol. *39:* 181–186 (1975).
9 Le Blanc, J.; Blais, B.; Barabé, B.; Côté, J.: Effects of temperature and wind on facial temperature, heart rate, and sensation. J. appl. Physiol. *40:* 127–131 (1976).
10 Hanna, J.N.; Hill, P.; Sinclair, J.D.: Human cardiorespiratory responses to acute cold exposure. Clin. exp. Pharmacol. Physiol. *2:* 229–238 (1975).
11 Raven, P.B.; Niki, I.; Dahms, T.E.; Horvath, S.M.: Compensatory cardiovascular responses during an environmental cold stress. J. appl. Physiol. *29:* 417–421 (1970).
12 Tabakin, B.S.; Hanson, J.S.; Merriam, T.W.; Caldwell, E.J.: Haemodynamic responses of normal men to graded exercise. J. appl. Physiol. *19:* 457–464 (1964).
13 Thauer, R.: Circulatory adjustments to climatic requirements; in Handbook of physiology, section 2, circulation, vol. 3, pp. 1921–1966 (American Physiological Society, Bethesda 1965).
14 Wilkerson, J.E.; Raven, P.B.; Bolduan, N.W.; Horvath, S.M.: Adaptation in man's adrenal function in response to acute cold stress. J. appl. Physiol. *36:* 183–189 (1974).
15 Keatinge, W.; Malcolm, B.; McIlory, B.; Goldfien, A.: Cardiovascular responses to ice-cold showers. J. appl. Physiol. *19:* 1145–1150 (1964).
16 Baur, W.F.: Über den Einfluss der äusseren Wärme und Kälte auf den lebenden menschlichen Körper (Marburg 1804).
17 Wayne, E.J.; Graybiel, A.: Observations on effect of food, gastric distension, external temperature, and repeated exercise on angina of effort, with note on angina sine dolore. Clin. Sci. *1:* 287–304 (1934).
18 Lassvik, C.T.; Areskog, N.-H.: Angina in cold environment. Reactions to exercise. Br. Heart J. *42:* 396–401 (1979).
19 Lassvik, C.T.; Areskog, N.-H.: Angina pectoris during inhalation of cold air. Reactions to exercise. Br. Heart J. *43:* 661–667 (1980).
20 Epstein, S.E.; Stampfer, M.; Beiser, G.D.; Goldstein, R.E.: Braunwald, E.: Effects of a reduction in environmental temperature on the circulatory response to exercise in man. Implications concerning angina pectoris. New Engl. J. Med. *280:* 7–11 (1969).
21 Neill, W.A.; Duncan, D.A.; Kloster, F.; Mahler, D.J.: Response of coronary circulation to cutaneous cold. Am. J. Med. *56:* 471–476 (1974).
22 Abboud, F.M.; Eckstein, J.W.: Reflex vasoconstrictor and vasodilator response in man. Circulation Res. *18/19:* suppl. 1, pp. 96–103 (1966).
23 Leon, D.F.; Amidi, M.; Leonard, J.J.: Left heart work and temperature responses to cold exposure in man. Am. J. Cardiol. *26:* 38–45 (1970).
24 Parry, C.H.: An inquiry into the symptoms and causes of the syncope anginosa commonly called angina pectoris. (Cruttwell, Bath 1799).

G. Prager, MD, Pfluggasse 1, D-8400 Regensburg (FRG)

Adv. Pharmacother., vol. 1, pp. 137–142 (Karger, Basel 1982)

Buccal Synchron Nitroglycerin in Acute Treatment of Angina pectoris Attacks

A Comparison with Sublingually Administered Nitroglycerin in Patients with Stable Coronary Artery Disease

Gerold Prager

Regensburg, FRG

Introduction

Ohlmeier [1] and *Langbehn* [2] have shown in hemodynamic studies that buccal administration of Synchron nitroglycerin affects the pulmonary artery pressure in a way comparable to the effects after sublingual administration of nitroglycerin. The systolic, diastolic, and mean pulmonary pressures were significantly reduced at 30 s after buccal administration of 1, 2.5, and 5 mg Synchron nitroglycerin. Therefore, the purpose of our study was to investigate whether buccally administered Synchron nitroglycerin could not only be used for acute and long-term prophylaxis, but also for acute treatment of angina pectoris attacks, and the relief of anginal attacks by buccal administration of Synchron nitroglycerin tablets (2.5 mg) in comparison with sublingually administered nitroglycerin capsules (0.8 mg) under normal conditions.

Methods

Selection of Patients and Study Design

11 patients with stable coronary heart disease documented by exercise testing were instructed to relieve any anginal attack by buccal administration of Synchron nitroglycerin or sublingual administration of nitroglycerin capsules on 2 different study days. Among 11 patients admitted to the study, 2 patients had no anginal episodes during the study phase, and 1 was excluded because of wrong drug application (simultaneous administration of capsule and tablet). Thus, data sets of 8 patients (6 males and 2 females) were statistically evaluated. The average age of this group was 56.7 years, ranging from 41 to 66 years.

The buccally administered nitroglycerin tablet was positioned in the lower pouch of the cheek, the nitroglycerin capsule chewed and sublingually positioned for fast absorption. All patients were trained in the handling of a stopwatch to avoid measuring errors.

Measurement Parameters

During the 2 subsequent test phases each patient recorded the following target variables in connection with relief of anginal attacks: (1) the interval between application of test drug and onset of action (measured by stopwatch) and (2) the total duration of anginal attack (also measured by stopwatch). All data were documented in a patient protocol. Furthermore, each patient was interviewed about his subjective impression regarding the efficacy of the two test agents.

Statistical Analysis

Individual measurements of each patient were used to compute intraindividual data per test phase. Then all individual measurements of the total population during one test phase were calculated as the total (weighted) mean value. The resulting standard deviation consists of the intraindividual as well as the interindividual component of variation.

The subsequent statistical analysis of target variables using the paired t test required the calculation of differences between the intraindividual mean values of the two test phases. In line with the medical model the zero hypothesis had to be tested, saying: the average difference between the test agents does not differ from zero ($H_0{:}\mu d = 0$).

Results

The individual frequencies of anginal attacks are summarized in table I. The difference between the two test drug groups is not statistically significant.

Onset of Action

The interval in seconds between application of each test substance and the onset of action is presented as intraindividual mean values in table II.

After buccal administration of Synchron nitroglycerin, the onset of action occurs on average at 84.0 s, after sublingually administered nitroglycerin at 63.3 s. The difference is statistically significant ($p < 0.01$), however, with a high standard deviation of 66.9 or 64.8. Patient No. 6 showed extraordinary average values of 4 min after both test drugs, evidently based on patient-specific causes. A similar but less pronounced effect at 2 min was observed in patient No. 8, however, on the basis of only one or two anginal attacks. Eliminating these two extreme values the interindividual mean value is reduced by about 30% to approximately 40 s after nitroglycerin administered sublingually. After buccal application of Synchron nitroglycerin, the total mean is reduced to about 1 min, again excluding the two extreme values of patients No. 6 and 8 which hardly affected the difference between the two test agents.

Table I. Individual frequencies of anginal attacks

Patient No.	Phase I sublingually administered nitroglycerin capsules	Phase II buccally administered Synchron nitroglycerin tablets
1	6	12
2	8	3
3	4	5
4	4	6
5	5	7
6	3	4
7	2	2
8	1	2
Mean value	4.1	5.1
Median	4.0	4.5
Minimum	1	2
Maximum	8	12

Table II. Interval (s) between application and onset of action

Patient No.	Phase I sublingually administered nitroglycerin capsules	Phase II buccally administered Synchron nitroglycerin tablets	Difference phase II–I
1	41.7	53.7	12.0
2	45.1	77.3	32.2
3	35.0	51.2	16.2
4	53.0	91.8	38.8
5	41.4	47.3	5.9
6	250.0	259.2	9.2
7	20.0	32.0	12.0
8	130.0	165.0	35.0
Mean value	63.3[1]	84.0[1]	20.2[2]
Standard deviation	64.8	66.9	13.0
Minimum	16	23	5.9
Maximum	285	291	38.8

[1] Calculated from all individual measurements ('weighted mean').
[2] Calculated from the differences of intraindividual mean values; $p < 0.01$ with $t = 4.38$. DF = 7 (paired Student t test).

Duration of Attacks

The duration of anginal attacks in seconds after respective relief is presented as intraindividual mean values in table III.

The average duration of anginal attacks amounts to 6.5 min after buccal application of Synchron nitroglycerin and to 5 min after sublingual administration. The difference between the two drugs is not statistically significant. In patients No. 4 and 6 the duration of anginal attacks is reduced by more than 2 min or 0.5 min after buccal application of nitroglycerin compared with the sublingually administered capsule.

Subjective Impression of the Patients

Asked about their subjective feelings, 5 patients assessed the onset of action after sublingual administration of nitroglycerin capsules as being faster than that after the buccally administered Synchron nitroglycerin tablet. 2 patients considered both drugs equivalent, and 1 patient felt to be the buccally administered tablet superior to the sublingually administered capsule.

Table III. Duration (s) of anginal attacks

Patient No.	Phase I sublingually administered nitroglycerin capsules	Phase II buccally administered nitroglycerin tablets	Difference phase II–I
1	500.0	630.0	130.0
2	95.1	133.3	38.2
3	57.5	91.0	33.5
4	843.5	713.2	–130.3
5	74.6	90.4	15.8
6	360.0	330.0	– 30.0
7	270.0	330.0	60.0
8	480.0	540.0	60.0
Mean value	298.1[1]	387.9[1]	22.2[2]
Standard deviation	295.7	290.2	76.4
Minimum	45	74	–130.3
Maximum	1,292	913	130.0

[1] Calculated from all individual measurements ('weighted mean').

[2] Calculated from the differences of intraindividual mean values; not significant with t = 0.82, DF = 7 (paired Student t test).

Discussion and Conclusion

During the two test phases, 74 attacks of angina pectoris were documented. Among these, 41 anginal attacks were treated with buccally administered Synchron nitroglycerin tablets and 33 cases with nitroglycerin capsules for sublingual administration. The relief of attacks was observed in all 74 cases, i.e., there was no therapy failure.

After sublingual application of nitroglycerin, the onset of action occurred on average at 63 s, after buccally administered Synchron nitroglycerin at 84 s. Though the difference between the two test groups is statistically significant, it is of no clinical relevance because of high interindividual variation.

Since, according to *Davis* [3], the dissolution rate of the buccally administered tablet and, thus, also of the initial absorption rate, depends on saliva secretion at the site of application, the reason for the somewhat slower onset of action after buccally administered tablets may partly be due to the site. The patient-specific differences in behavior influencing the subjective criterion of anginal chest pain should be noted.

While the different hemodynamic parameters measured to demonstrate the onset of action under laboratory conditions showed only minor mean value variations after nitrate application [1, 2, 4–6], the effect on the subjective onset of action and the duration of anginal attack shows considerable individual variations under clinical conditions.

The present study demonstrates that buccally administered Synchron nitroglycerin tablets are suitable for acute treatment of anginal attacks. Since buccal, controlled release nitroglycerin can be applied for acute and long-term prophylaxis due to its prolonged drug release properties, any double application of nitroglycerin in various formulations can be discarded in patients with coronary artery disease.

References

1 Ohlmeier, H.; Mertens, H.M.; Mannebach, H.; Gleichmann, U.: The effect of buccal Synchron nitroglycerin on pulmonary artery pressure: a comparison with sublingual nitroglycerin in patients with coronary heart disease (in this book).

2 Langbehn, A.-F.; Beurich, H.W.; Leupold, H.; Hoffmann, R.; Sheikhzaden, A.; Lohaus, R.: Effect of buccal synchron nitroglycerin on pulmonary artery pressure at rest and during exercise. A comparison with sublingual nitroglycerin in patients with coronary artery disease (in this book).

3 Davis, S.S.; Daly, P.B.; Kennerley, J.W.; Frier, M.; Hardy, J.G.; Wilson, C.G.: Design and evaluation of sustained release formulations for oral and buccal administration (in this book).

4 Grüntzig, A.: Wirkungseintritt des Isosorbiddinitrat-Sprays. 2. Nitrat-Symposion, Berlin 1980, pp. 403–405.

5 Niederer, W., et al.: Wirkungsnachweis von ISDN-Spray am Ventrikulogramm bei koronarer Herzerkrankung. 2. Nitrat-Symposion, Berlin 1980, pp. 146–149.

6 Simon, H., et al.; Nichtinvasive Nachweismethoden zur Akutwirkung von Nitroverbindungen auf das Myokard bei koronarer Herzerkrankung. 2. Nitroglycerin-Symposion, Hamburg 1979, pp. 29–44.

G. Prager, MD, Pfluggasse 1, D-8400 Regensburg (FRG)

Discussion

Chairman: *W.-D. Bussmann*

Langbehn: Concerning the question whether buccally administered Synchron nitroglycerin is effective in acute anginal attacks, I would like to report some of our own findings. In 16 of 19 patients the anginal attack was successfully treated with 2.5 mg of buccal nitroglycerin. The symptoms subsided after an average time of 83 s. This demonstrates that buccally administered nitroglycerin can be used as a rapid antianginal drug.

Gleichmann: Dr. *Prager,* you extensively discussed the point of possible vasospasm as a cause of cold-induced angina. But I am not yet convinced that vasospasm does not play a role in your patients. First of all, we know from the work of *Maseri* that you may have ST segment depression in cases with vasospasms. When there are no major vessels involved then you may have ST segment depression. Secondly, from your figure we can see that in the patient with cold-induced angina, there is a heart rate increase and ST segment depression too after buccal application. My interpretation would be that in spite of this increase we have less vasospasm, and so the patient does not get his angina.

Prager: The long-term ECG did not give any hint of coronary artery spasm inducing angina pectoris, demonstrated by the complete lack of ST segment elevations. It is well known that in patients with spontaneous angina pectoris, various ECG changes can be found: there may be isolated T wave alterations or isolated ST segment depressions. But my experience with spontaneous angina pectoris is that in addition to ST segment depression ST segment elevations always occur. The long-term ECG analysis system used in this study cannot differentiate between pathological, i.e., ascending ST segments, since the system has only one measuring point in the ST segment to compare changes with a reference point in the QRS complex.

Wagner: In your first study, the cold-induced study, you found a significant prolongation of the cold exposure interval. But you did not see a reduction in total number of attacks. Might this be due to the 1.0 mg buccal dosage, or do you have another explanation for that phenomenon?

Prager: The patient exercises up to the occurrence of symptoms, i.e., after nitroglycerin the patient continues to walk until symptoms occur, thus reaching a new, higher exercise tolerance. Therefore, the therapeutic success is not reflected in the frequency of anginal attacks but in the prolongation of cold exposure intervals.

Adv. Pharmacother., vol. 1, pp. 143–154 (Karger, Basel 1982)

Angina Prophylaxis with Buccal Synchron Nitroglycerin: A Rapid Onset Long-Acting Nitrate[1]

Nathaniel Reichek, Cheryl Priest, Michael Kienzle, Joseph P. Kleaveland, Sanford Bolton, Martin St. John Sutton

The Noninvasive Laboratory, Cardiovascular Section, Department of Medicine, University of Pennsylvania and the Hospital of the University of Pennsylvania and the College of Pharmacy and Allied Health Professions, St. John's University, Philadelphia, Pa., USA

The effectiveness of sublingual nitroglycerin (GTN) for prevention of exercise-induced angina pectoris is well documented [1]. While sublingual GTN is potent and has a rapid onset of action, detectible effects of angina prophylaxis are gone within 1 h of administration [4]. Therefore, numerous 'long-acting' nitrate preparations have been devised and employed clinically with the goal of providing sustained, predictable angina prophylaxis throughout have the day [2, 3]. However, none of the agents in clinical use has a time course of action and potency that is optimal for this purpose. For example, sublingual isosorbide dinitrate has a relatively rapid onset of effect but its duration of action is also short – perhaps no more than 1 h – when prevention of exertional angina is the end-point [4]. Oral and cutaneous nitrates have more prolonged effects, but onset of action is delayed and the magnitude of effect often smaller than that of sublingual GTN [5–7]. Moreover, the duration of anti-anginal effects beyond 3 h with oral and cutaneous nitrates is controversial. Recently, plethysmographic studies in normals have demonstrated that buccal administration of a sustained release GTN lozenge (buccal Synchron nitroglycerin = BGTN) can combine rapid onset of physiologic effect with duration of up to 6 h [8]. However, hemodynamic effects of nitrates often last longer than demonstrable anti-anginal efficacy [4]. Therefore, the present study was designed to determine the efficacy of BGTN in

[1] Supported by NIH 5 MO1 RR00040, by a Commonwealth of Pennsylvania Health Services Contract, and a grant from Forest Laboratories.

prevention of exercise-induced angina using a well characterized double-blind exercise protocol which has been used previously to evaluate many other nitrates [2].

Methods

Population. Studies were performed in 15 subjects, 14 male, ranging in age from 38 to 67 years. All had typical chronic stable exertional angina for at least 6 months prior to study. All had objective evidence of coronary artery disease consisting of prior documented myocardial infarction in 6, coronary angiography in 10, reversible perfusion defects on exercise thallium scans in 2 and exercise-induced segmental wall motion abnormality by two-dimensional echocardiography during upright exercise in 3. Angina was precipitated by treadmill exercise testing in all. 5 subjects had undergone prior coronary artery bypass surgery and had recurrent stable exertional angina. 14 were receiving propranolol in doses of 40–320 mg daily, mean dose 101.5 mg. 10 were receiving long-acting nitrates chronically prior to admission. Historical frequency of angina on these regimens ranged from 1 to 14 attacks per week.

Protocol. All subjects were admitted to an inpatient Clinical Research Center and underwent routine admission evaluation including detailed history, physical examination, electrocardiogram, chest roentgenogram, complete blood count, urinalysis, and a standard biochemical profile (SMA-12). All hematologic and biochemical data were normal save for persistant mild hyperglycemia in 1 subject due to maturation onset diabetes mellitus discovered during evaluation. Administration of propranolol and noncardiac medications, if any, was continued during the study. Long-acting nitrates were discontinued at admission and sublingual GTN provided for treatment of angina. Only 1 subject had spontaneous episodes of exertional angina during hospitalization, which were relieved by rest. An appropriate dose of BGTN was selected for each subject by serial administration of BGTN lozenges in doses of 1.0, 1.5, 2.0, 2.5 and 5.0 mg placed between the upper lip and gum as needed until a dose was identified which produced a consistent 10 mm Hg reduction in sitting blood pressure and/or a 10-beat per minute increase in heart rate. Each dose tested was administered on a different day, in the absence of other nitrates, after completion of practice exercise testing and a 30- to 60-min rest period. Blood pressure and heart rate were determined repeatedly with the subject sitting with legs dependent in a quiet environment prior to administration of each test dose of BGTN until stable values were obtained; then every 5 min for the first hour of administration and once hourly thereafter for 5 h if a response was seen in the first hour. The time to dissolution of the tablet was noted. The smallest dose of BGTN that produced the defined effects on heart rate and blood pressure was used for exercise studies. This procedure has been shown to reliably identify a nitrate dose that can produce anti-anginal prophylaxis [4, 5], and permits selection of physiologically comparable doses of any nitrate in each subject. Practice exercise tests were performed on the second and third day of hospitalization before, and 0.5, 1, 2, 3 and 5 h after administration of a known placebo, physically indistinguishable from BGTN. On days 4 and 5, placebo and active BGTN were administered, from blinded bottles of medication, based on tables of randomized sequence. Serial exercise tests were repeated as on days 2 and 3. On days 4 and 5, sublingual GTN in the subject's usual dose was also administered at 5.5 h after placebo and BGTN administration, respectively, and exercise repeated 3 min after administration.

Exercise Procedure. The National Heart Institute's bicycle ergometer protocol, a well-documented procedure used extensively in the past to evaluate nitrate anti-anginal effects, was used [1–4]. Briefly, an individualized sequence of workloads was selected for each subject so that, in the absence of an active nitrate, the onset of angina occurred during the second 3-min stage of exercise. Subjects pedalled a Godart constant load bicycle ergometer steadily at 40–50 revolutions per minute and workload was increased by 20 W every 3 min. Exercise was stopped and exercise duration recorded when angina onset occurred. A single-lead CM5 electrocardiogram was monitored continuously and recorded before and at 1-min intervals during exercise and recovery and heart rate, ST segment changes and arrhythmias, if any, noted. Blood pressure was recorded before, during and after exercise, with determinations at 2.5 min of exercise and at 1-min intervals during and after the second and any subsequent stages. Room temperature was maintained constant at 72 °F and the time of exercise bouts and medication administration held constant on the blinded test days. The first two exercise bouts each day were performed in the fasting state but a clear fluid breakfast was ingested after the 1-hour post-medication exercise bout and a full fluid lunch provided after the 3-hour bout. In 2 subjects who were unrepentant cigarette smokers, care was taken to assure that smoking occurred at the same time and the same number of cigarettes were consumed on the two test days. The time of complete dissolution of the buccal lozenge was noted on each day.

Statistical Analyses. At the end of the study, the blinding sequence was decoded and two-way analysis of variance was used to compare values for heart rate, blood pressure, ST segment change, work load and exercise duration before and after placebo and BGTN, and heart rate and blood pressure responses to BGTN test doses at rest. Sublingual GTN tests were compared by paired t-test. Qualitative differences between BGTN and placebo, such as whether exercise ended with fatigue or angina, were compared using the sign test.

Results

The dose of BGTN required to affect upright resting heart rate and/or blood pressure ranged from 1.0 to 2.5 mg with a mean of 1.6 mg. The time course of heart rate and blood pressure after administration of the selected dose of BGTN is shown in figure 1. Significant reductions in blood pressure were present at 5 min and persisted for 2 h, but individual responses were quite variable in duration. In contrast, heart rate showed no significant changes, perhaps because of the substantial doses of propranolol taken by most subjects. On the blinded test days (4 and 5) placebo was administered first in 7 subjects and BGTN first in 8.

The reproducibility of the onset of angina with this study design is evident from the stability of exercise duration to angina on the blinded placebo test day (fig. 2). The similarity of the pre-medication control exercise durations on day 4 and 5 (fig. 3a) also demonstrates this. In the absence of an active nitrate no significant alteration of exercise duration occurred. After

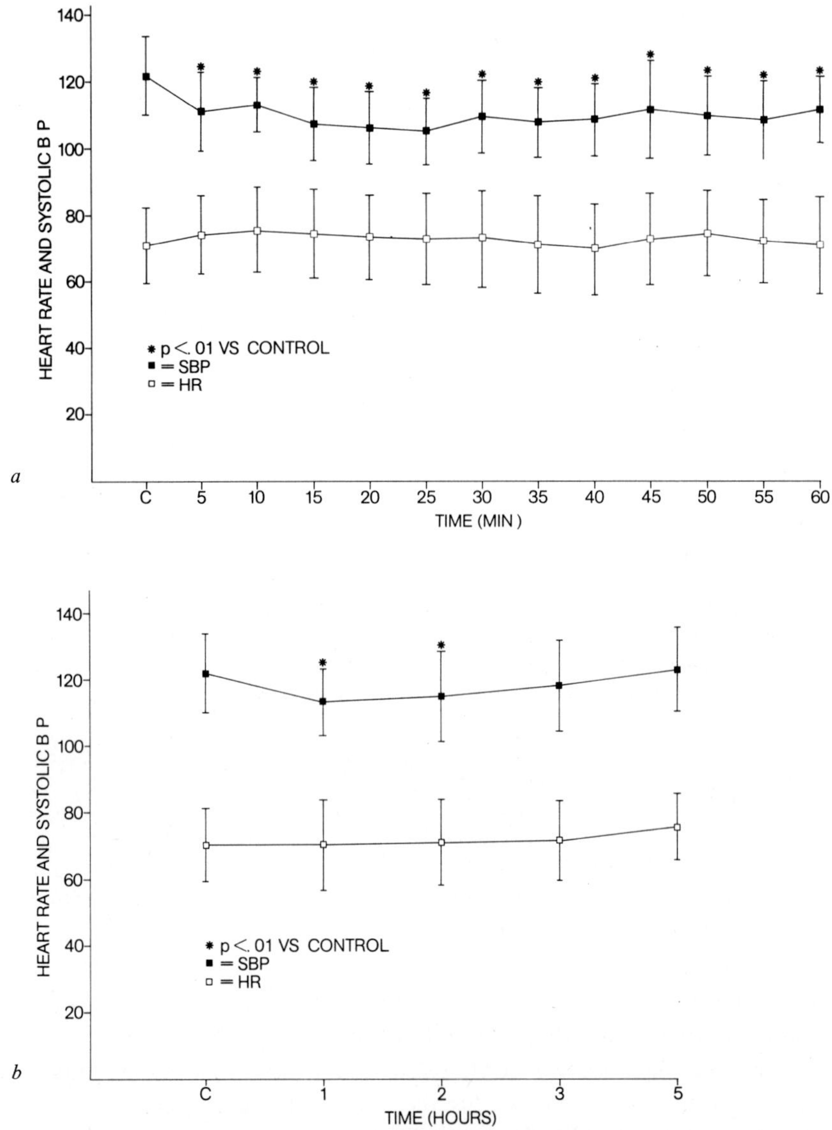

Fig. 1. *a* Time course of resting heart rate (HR) and systolic blood pressure (SBP) before (C = control) and for 1 h after administration of BGTN in each subject. Means for the group with 1 SD are shown. Heart rate does not change significantly but systolic blood pressure falls significantly within 5 min and remains lower than control throughout. *b* Time course of HR and SBP over 5 h after BGTN. SBP is significantly below control for 2 h.

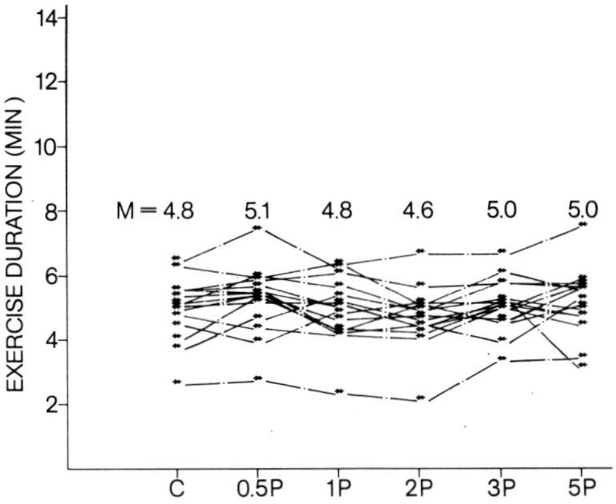

Fig. 2. Duration of premedication control exercise bout (C) on placebo test day compared with exercise duration at 0.5–5 h after placebo (P). No placebo effect is evident, exercise duration varies little in individual subjects, and all mean values are very similar.

placebo, all bouts of exercise except one (subject 13, 1 h past placebo) ended with angina.

In contrast, the effect of BGTN, as compared to placebo, on exercise duration at 0.5 h after administration is shown in figure 3b. Mean exercise duration increased from 5.1 to 7.3 min ($p < 0.01$), with improvement of more than 1 min in 13 of 15 subjects. Moreover, 7 of 15 subjects terminated exercise because of fatigue rather than angina ($p < 0.05$), and angina occurred at a higher workload in 6 of 15 subjects ($p < 0.05$). Similarly, significant prolongation of exercise duration was seen at 1, 2, 3 and 5 h after BGTN (fig. 3c–f, table I). Exercise to fatigue occurred in 8 subjects at 1 h ($p < 0.05$), 4 at 2 h, 4 at 3 h and 3 at 5 h. Increase in workload at angina occurred in 3 at 1 h, 7 at 2 h ($p < 0.05$), 4 at 3 h and 5 at 5 h. ST segment changes at angina, and duration of angina were similar throughout on BGTN and placebo days. However, ST segment depression at the same workload prior to angina fell from 1.8 mm on placebo to 1.2 mm on BGTN ($n = 59$, $p < 0.001$).

The relative peak effects of BGTN and sublingual GTN can be examined by comparison of exercise duration after BGTN at the time of its peak effect as compared to that found 3 min after administration of sublingual GTN. Figure 4 shows the maximal exercise duration at any time after BGTN administration plotted against that after sublingual GTN and reveals that BGTN and sublingual GTN had comparable peak effects, with mean

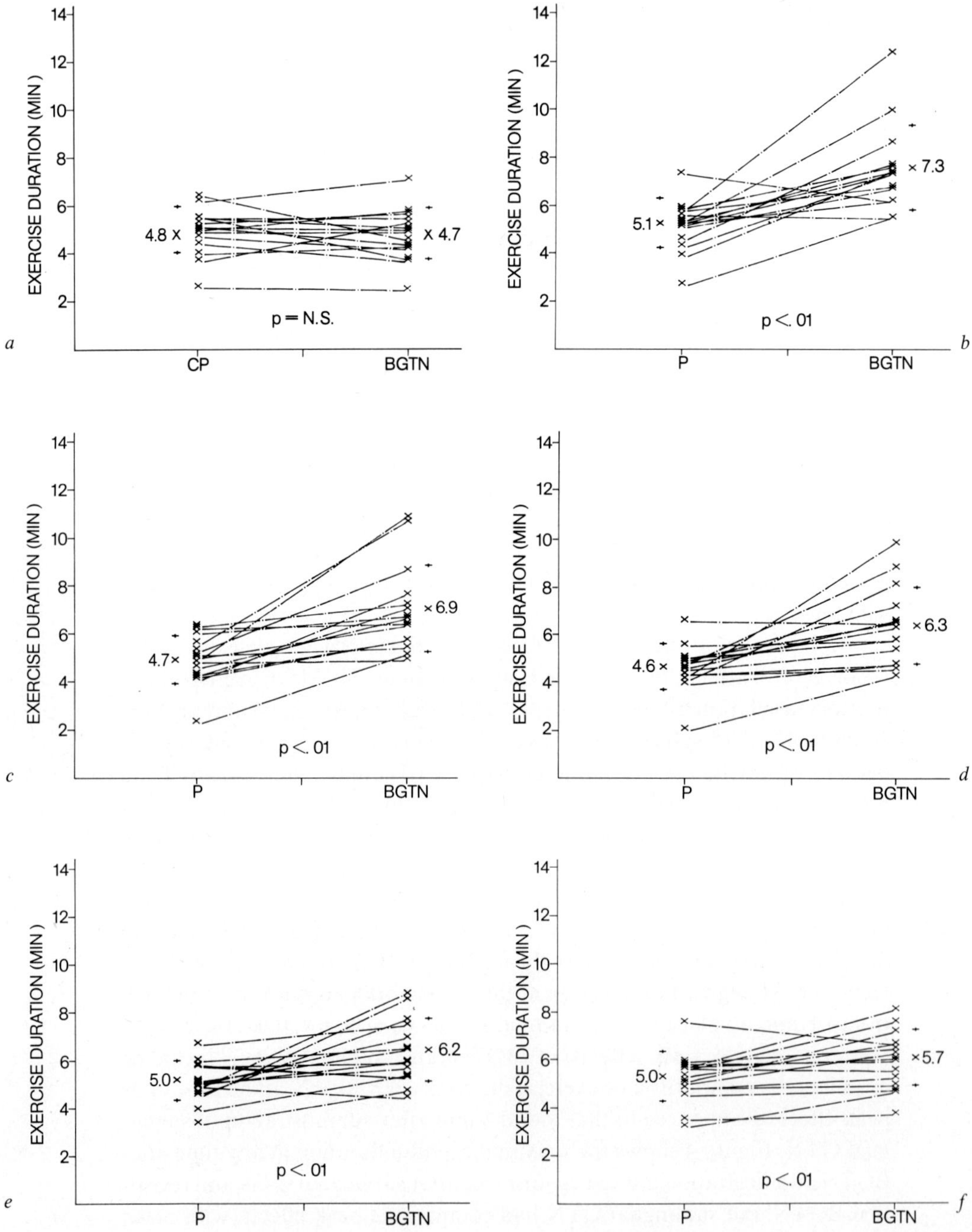
EXERCISE DURATION (MIN)
14
12
10
8
6
4
2
4.8 ×
× 4.7
p = N.S.
CP
BGTN
a
5.1 ×
× 7.3
p < .01
P
BGTN
b
4.7 ×
× 6.9
p < .01
c
4.6 ×
× 6.3
p < .01
d
5.0 ×
× 6.2
p < .01
e
5.0 ×
× 5.7
p < .01
f

Table I. Exercise duration before and after placebo (P) and buccal nitroglycerin (BGTN)

Subject	Agent	Control	0.5 h	1 h	2 h	3 h	5 h	GTN
1	P	4.6	4.2	4.0	3.9	4.8	4.3	7.7
	BGTN	4.1	7.1	7.5	4.7	4.3	4.5	7.5
2	P	4.3	3.8	4.7	5.0	5.0	3.0	7.9
	BGTN	3.6	7.2	4.8	5.7	6.3	4.4	7.9
3	P	5.0	5.2	4.5	4.6	4.5	5.4	7.5
	BGTN	4.9	7.5	6.5	6.5	7.5	7.3	–
4	P	4.8	5.2	4.1	4.3	3.8	5.1	4.2
	BGTN	4.8	6.0	5.6	4.5	5.2	6.4	4.1
5	P	5.4	5.5	4.9	4.3	5.0	4.6	6.5
	BGTN	5.0	5.3	6.2	4.7	5.5	5.0	6.0
6	P	4.9	5.0	5.0	4.5	4.9	5.7	6.5
	BGTN	5.7	6.5	5.3	5.3	5.8	6.2	6.7
7	P	5.4	5.3	4.9	4.3	4.8	5.5	11.4
	BGTN	3.7	9.7	10.7	9.7	8.6	7.8	15.4
8	P	3.6	4.5	5.2	4.8	5.6	5.5	8.5
	BGTN	5.2	8.4	8.5	6.2	5.1	5.8	9.2
9	P	5.0	5.8	5.5	4.8	5.1	4.8	12.4
	BGTN	4.3	12.1	10.5	8.7	4.8	6.0	11.3
10	P	3.9	5.1	4.2	4.9	4.4	4.9	7.6
	BGTN	4.2	7.1	6.9	7.1	8.3	6.9	–
11	P	6.3	7.2	6.1	5.0	5.9	5.4	6.3
	BGTN	4.5	6.0	6.3	6.4	6.3	5.3	6.6
12	P	5.4	5.7	5.9	5.5	5.6	5.6	7.0
	BGTN	5.4	6.6	6.6	5.7	5.7	5.7	6.2
13	P	6.1	5.8	6.2	6.5	6.5	7.3	7.6
	BGTN	7.0	7.4	7.1	6.4	7.3	6.4	7.0
14	P	2.5	2.6	2.2	2.0	3.2	3.3	6.8
	BGTN	2.4	5.3	5.0	4.2	4.6	3.5	6.7
15	P	5.2	5.3	4.2	4.1	4.9	4.6	8.3
	BGTN	5.6	7.2	5.6	8.0	6.8	4.7	8.8
Mean	P	4.8	5.1	4.7	4.6	5.0	5.0	7.7
	BGTN	4.7	7.3*	6.9*	6.3*	6.2*	5.7*	7.9

*$p < 0.01$ vs placebo.

Fig. 3. *a* Exercise duration on control bouts before placebo (P) and before BGTN is quite similar. *b* Exercise duration 0.5 h after P and BGTN in 15 subjects. A significant increase in mean exercise duration of 2.2 min occurs after BGTN, with improvement of more than 1 min in 13/15. *c* Exercise duration 1 h after P or BGTN. Mean duration is significantly increased from 4.7 to 6.9 min. *d* Exercise duration 2 h after P and BGTN. Mean exercise duration increases significantly by 1.7 min. *e* Exercise duration 3 h after P or BGTN. Exercise duration increases significantly after BGTN by 1.2 min. *f* Exercise duration 5 h after P or BGTN. Duration increases significantly by 0.7 min after BGTN.

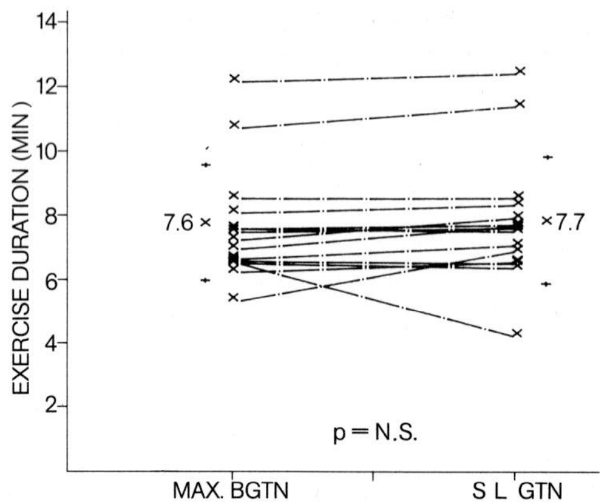

Fig. 4. Exercise duration after sublingual GTN and at maximal BGTN effect in each subject. Mean values do not differ significantly.

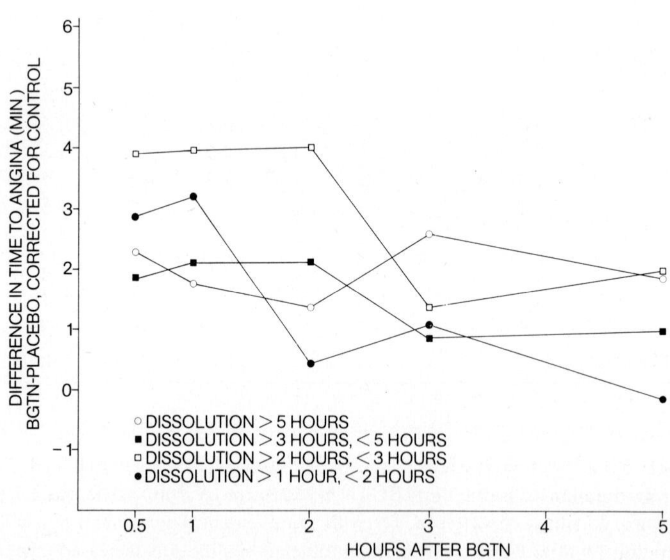

Fig. 5. Relationship of BGTN dissolution time to magnitude of exercise prolongation relative to placebo at a given time after BGTN administration. A plateau effect is present so long as the tablet is physically present.

exercise duration of 7.6 and 7.7 min, respectively. 8 subjects exercised to exhaustion after BGTN as compared to 8 after sublingual GTN. Maximal exercise tolerance was also similar when sublingual GTN was administered after BGTN and after placebo (7.9 vs 7.8 min).

The duration of BGTN effect bore a predictable relationship to the physical disappearance of the tablet from the buccal cavity. Figure 5 shows the mean prolongation of exercise duration by BGTN at each time tested for subgroups of subjects with dissolution in less than 2, 2–3, 3–5, and more than 5 h, respectively. A uniform plateau effect was evident in subjects whose tablet did not completely dissolve until after the 5-hour exercise test, while a plateau was observed in other subjects only for as long as the tablet was physically present. Conversely, dissolution within 3 h was associated with larger inital effects at 0.5 and 1 h.

BGTN did not produce severe headache in any individual, although 4 subjects had histories of inability to tolerate oral isosorbide dinitrate because of headache. A mild tingling or burning sensation on the buccal mucosa was noted immediately after administration but was not unpleasant. Symptomatic orthostatic hypotension did not occur. Presence of the tablet was not annoying to subjects and did not interfere with eating, drinking or conversation. 12 subjects noted a sense of 'fullness of the head', or similar sensations but this did not become unpleasant or impair ability to function.

Discussion

An ideal agent for prophylaxis of exertional angina should combine rapid onset, prolonged duration, potent effects, and the opportunity to titrate dose size and frequency easily so that an optimal regimen can be constructed for each patient. The data obtained in the present study suggest that BGTN has many of these characteristics. The time course of changes in upright blood pressure indicates onset of maximal hemodynamic effect within 5 min, while enhancement of exercise tolerance persists for up to 5 h. Since the same study design has been used repeatedly in the past to evaluate sublingual GTN, sublingual and oral isosorbide dinitrate and GTN ointment against placebo, it is possible to compare the time course of BGTN to that of these other commonly used agents [4–6]. With respect to onset of action, sublingual GTN produces hemodynamic effects within 2–3 min. In contrast, effects of sublingual isosorbide are first evident at 10 min. Other agents show more prolonged delays – on the order of 30–45 min for oral isosorbide dinitrate and cutaneous nitroglycerin. Thus BGTN may be preferable to agents other than sublingual GTN in speed of onset. The possibility also exists that BGTN may act as fast as sublingual GTN itself, offering the prospect of a single agent that could provide both rapid relief of an established episode of angina and sustained prophylaxis thereafter.

Similarly, no other 'long-acting' nitrate has been shown to have effects on exercise tolerance out to 5 h using this method of dose selection and this exercise protocol design. Sublingual isosorbide effects have lasted for 1 h or less, while cutaneous GTN and oral isosorbide have been shown to be effective only out to 3 h after administration. While the magnitude and consistency of buccal GTN's effect are less at 3 and 5 h than at 0.5–2 h, a similar pattern has been shown at 3 h with oral isosorbide dinitrate. The maximal effect obtained with BGTN is similar to that of sublingual GTN, sublingual and oral isosorbide dinitrate and cutaneous GTN. Because of rapid onset combined with prolonged duration, the total duration of prophylaxis obtained with a single dose of BGTN is up to 5 h. In contrast, because of delayed onset, the total duration of cutaneous GTN effect for prophylaxis of angina may last only 2 h, from 1 to 3 h after administration. Similarly, the total duration of oral isosorbide dinitrate effect may be only 2 h (from 1 to 3 h after administration) and that of sublingual isosorbide only 50 min, when assessed by the methods used in this study. One recent report by *Thadani* et al. [9] describes enhanced effort tolerance with oral isosorbide dinitrate lasting for 8 h. However, none of those subjects were beta-blocked, whereas all subjects in the present study were receiving full doses of propranolol. Thus, we compared exercise tolerance on propranolol plus placebo to that on propranolol plus BGTN, whereas they compared exercise tolerance on no active agent to exercise tolerance on isosorbide. This may magnify the apparent isosorbide effect. Moreover, the blood pressure change observed by *Thadani* et al. [9] on the smallest dose tested was four times what we observed, so that the relative dose used was much larger than the ones we tested. Such large doses may not be well tolerated in beta-blocked patients.

A fundamental problem in design of optimal nitrate regimens for angina prophylaxis is the inherent variability of dose-response relationships and duration of action in different individuals of all nitrates that have been evaluated to date. BGTN has several characteristics that might simplify the problem. It has been shown repeatedly that a nitrate dose sufficient to produce an orthostatic fall in blood pressure and/or increase in heart rate, with any preparation, will produce some demonstrable enhancement of exercise tolerance [1–3]. This relationship can be used to identify an initial minimal dose of nitrate that will be both safe, and at least somewhat effective, although subsequent dose increments may also be needed in clinical use. Unfortunately, for most 'long-acting' nitrates, slow onset of action makes dose titration with pulse and blood pressure determinations impractical in the clinical setting. The rapid onset of BGTN effect may obviate this problem. Within 10 min of administration, presence or absence of orthostatic effect is amply documented, so that dose titration is practical in the outpatient setting. In addition, the patient can determine readily whether the tablet has dissolved or not. Since the time course of BGTN effect is determined by the time to tablet dissolution, dose frequency can be established based on the patient's observations on duration of dissolution and timing of symptoms. Angina occurring while the tablet is still present might be an indication for a dose increase, while symptoms occurring between the time of tablet dissolution and the next dose would be an indication for a shorter dose interval. Initial experience with chronic administration in 9 patients suggests that this approach will be useful. Finally, beyond the properties of present BGTN tablets, the inherent design characteristics of the system offer great flexibility in creation of additional preparations to meet specific needs. Thus, BGTN may have the capacity to become an ideal system for chronic administration of GTN.

Acknowledgements

We are deeply indebted to *Theodore Plappert* and *Ali Muhammad* for their assistance in statistical analysis, to Ms. *Lesly Stalford* for administrative support, to Mrs. *Patricia Wyatt* for manuscript preparation, to Dr. *Joseph Schor* and Mr. *Howard Solomon* of Forest Laboratories for the opportunity to perform this project, and to Dr. *John A. Kastor*, Chief, Cardiovascular Section, for his encouragement and assistance.

References

1 Goldstein, R.E.; Epstein, S.E.: Nitrates in the prophylactic treatment of angina pectoris. Circulation *48:* 917–920 (1973).

2 Russek, H.I.: Therapeutic role of coronary vasodilators: glyceryl trinitrate, isosorbide dinitrate and pentaerythritol tetranitrate. Am. J. med. Sci. *252:* 9–19 (1966).

3 Aronow, W.S.; Cheslun, H.M.: Sublingual isosorbide dinitrate therapy versus sublingual placebo in angina pectoris. Circulation *41:* 869–874 (1970).

4 Goldstein, R.E.; Rosing, D.R.; Redwood, D.R.; Beiser, G.D.; Epstein, S.E.: Clinical and circulatory effects of isosorbide dinitrate. Circulation *43:* 629–640 (1971).

5 Reichek, N.; Goldstein, R.E.; Redwood, D.R.; Epstein, S.E.: Sustained effects of nitroglycerin ointment in patients with angina pectoris. Circulation *50:* 348–352 (1974).

6 Danahy, D.T.; Burwell, D.T.; Aronow, W.S.; Prakash, R.: Sustained hemodynamic and antianginal effect of high dose oral isosorbide dinitrate. Circulation *55:* 381–387 (1977).
7 Markis, J.E.; Gorlin, R.; Mills, R.M.; Williams, R.A.; Schweitzer, P.; Ransil, B.J.: Sustained effect of orally administered isosorbide dinitrate on exercise performance of patients with angina pectoris. Am. J. Cardiol. *43:* 265–271 (1979).
8 Smolen, V.: Unpublished data.
9 Thadani, U.; Fung, H.; Darke, A.C.; Parker, J.O.: Oral isosorbide dinitrate in the treatment of angina pectoris: dose-response relationship and duration of action during acute therapy. Circulation *62:* 491–502 (1980).

N. Reichek, MD, Hospital of the University of Pennsylvania, 951 Gates,
3400 Spruce Street, Philadelphia, PA 19104 (USA)

Discussion

Chairmen: *U. Gleichmann* and *N. Reichek*

Békés: It might be that there is a so-called training effect, since you exercised the patient seven times.

Reichek: If one looks over the entire period of exercise, which is a 4-day program, there is a small training effect from the first to the second and sometimes the third exercise. Thereafter we are unable to show any training effect. If you recall one of the slides showing exercise duration before placebo and before buccal nitroglycerin on the third and fourth day, there is no training effect with this design. In part this may be related to the duration of the exercise which is very short.

Bussmann: Dr. *Ohlmeier* used in his study 2.5 mg buccal nitroglycerin and he observed effects for up to 3 h, but not longer. You described the effects of a smaller dose for up to 5 h. Might this not depend on the protocol – submaximal and maximal work load? The results might be influenced by a pretreatment with beta-blocking drugs.

Reichek: And virtually all these patients were very heavily beta-blockaded at the time of study. The results may look different with less or no beta-blockade but the other studies which have been done by this design would suggest that the conclusions about duration of action would not be affected by that difference. I think that this is an exquisitely sensitive study design, and that accounts for the differences in the durations reported.

Adv. Pharmacother., vol. 1, pp. 155–165 (Karger, Basel 1982)

Long-Term Buccal Administration of Synchron Nitroglycerin

N. Reichek, Ch.J. Priest, Martin St. John Sutton
Hospital of the University of Pennsylvania, Philadelphia, Pa., USA

Introduction

The purpose of this open-label, uncontrolled trial was to develop experience with outpatient use of buccally administered nitroglycerin to establish guidelines for clinical use.

Patients and Methods

Patient Selection

22 patients, 20 males and 2 females, ranging in age from 39 to 69 years, were enrolled. All had chronic stable angina at intake with objective laboratory documentation of coronary artery disease consisting of prior coronary angiography (16), documented prior infarction (9), exercise stress testing (9), or thallium or two-dimensional echocardiographic stress test showing segmental abnormality (6). 5 had undergone prior coronary bypass surgery. 8 had prior history of nitrate intolerance due to headache, and 1 patient could not tolerate propranolol well. The frequency of angina attacks by history at intake ranged from 'occasional' to 21 per week.

Methods

A series of outpatient visits over a 4-week period was utilized to assess patient responses to buccally administered nitroglycerin. The intake evaluation included a history and physical examination, electrocardiogram, chest X-ray, complete blood count, and a standard biochemical profile (SMA_{12}). 12 patients had been using long-acting nitrates which were tapered and discontinued during a lead-in period of 1 or 2 weeks. 15 patients were receiving propranolol which was continued.

The initial dose selection was accomplished by identifying the dose of nitroglycerin to be administered buccally which produced a fall in sitting blood pressure of 10 mm Hg or more and/or an increase in pulse rate of 10 beats/min or more. The starting dose after the titration ranged from 1.0 to 5.0 mg (mean 1.8 mg). The initial dose frequency was 1 tablet every 6 h, i.e., three times a day. The patients returned daily for 3 subsequent days after titration and once a week thereafter for evaluation and appropriate dose adjustment. The extension of the study was arranged with continued weekly outpatient visits if additional dose adjustment was necessary. 16 dose adjustments were performed during the treatment. In 3 cases the dose was reduced because of headache, in 9 cases the dose was increased because effort angina was not entirely eliminated with the tablet in place, in 2 cases the dose frequency was increased because of effort angina at times when the tablet had dissolved and the next dose was not yet due, and in three instances both dose size and frequency were increased to eliminate angina. Repeat electrocardiogram, chest X-ray, and blood studies were performed on all patients at the end of the 4-week period.

Results

20 patients completed the 1-month trial and there were 2 dropouts. 1 dropout occurred early in our experience, during slow progressive dose adjustment. The patient, a traveling businessman, felt his work did not permit the time necessary to reach the effective prophylactic level. We subsequently found that it was possible to increase the dose size and frequency over a period of several days to 1 week in order to avoid long periods of suboptimal therapy. The 2nd dropout could not tolerate other long-acting nitrates because of headache. He had previously tolerated up to 2 mg buccally administered nitroglycerin during a single-dose inpatient exercise study, but during this present study developed unacceptable headaches on 1 mg and was dropped.

Of the 20 subjects completing the study, the frequency of anginal attacks decreased in all but 1 patient. This individual, who had undergone coronary bypass surgery and had patent grafts, was subsequently hospitalized for persistent pain at rest which proved refractory to high-dose oral nitrates, cutaneous nitroglycerin, and propranolol. Despite the well-documented exercise-induced angina with ECG and the thallium scan abnormalities, it was not clear that all of her symptoms were in fact cardiac in origin. 10 subjects were entirely painfree at the end of 1 month of treatment. Even in those subjects where angina was not entirely eliminated, improvement was sometimes dramatic with anginal episodes in some cases decreasing from 15–16/week to 'occasional'.

Observations during the trial included complaint of initial headache (11 subjects), generally mild, which disappeared after a few days of use of buccally administered nitroglycerin. The estimated time of tablet dissolution ranged from 1 to 7 h, with a mean of 4.3 h. An increased dissolution rate occurred during prolonged physical activity, but dissolution rate tended to decline with experience. We believe this was due to patients' learning not to manipulate the tablet with their tongues.

A few subjects noted a burning sensation, which they also got with sublingually administered nitroglycerin, at the tablet site at study onset, but this did not persist. 17 patients showed mild and transient injection, due to local vasodilation at the site of tablet application. 4 patients showed initially mild erythema. Vasodilation and erythema diminished with continued use. There were no other local effects. 17 of 20 subjects completing the trial elected to continue using buccally administered nitroglycerin and have continued to do so. 9 patients with more severe and frequent angina use it on a regular schedule 3–4 times a day. 8 patients with less severe angina prefer to use it on a pro re nata basis for angina prophylaxis. Although advised not to do so, 3 subjects substituted the buccal for sublingual preparation of nitroglycerin for relief of angina at times and reported that it was as effective or more effective than the sublingual preparation. For detailed general data, see Appendix.

Discussion

While this is not a controlled trial, we have previously documented the ability of buccally administered nitroglycerin to enhance the effort tolerance for up to 5 h in a blinded, crossover, placebo-controlled trial. Our impression based on the clinical experience of outpatient use of buccally administered nitroglycerin is that it appears superior to other available long-acting nitrates in terms of efficacy, acceptability to patients, and ease of titration. We have the strong impression that it is tolerated without headache by many individuals who are otherwise unable to use long-acting nitrates and believe this may be due to the lack of dumping and even, continued protection provided by the preparation. It is striking that the total amount of administered nitroglycerin per 24 h required for control of angina is much lower than with other long-acting nitroglycerin preparations. This may indicate that a higher proportion of administered nitroglycerin arrives at target sites as the intact molecule rather than as a metabolite. It is known that nitroglycerin is more potent than its metabolites.

It is noteworthy that there was no change in ECG or laboratory findings as determined by repeat ECG and SMA_{12} after 1 month of the study.

N. Reichek, MD, Hospital of the University of Pennsylvania, 3400 Spruce Street, Philadelphia, PA 19104 (USA)

Appendix. Controlled-release study on bucally administered nitroglycerin – outpatient data

Patient No.	Age years	Sex	Diagnosis	Medication	Prior nitrates	Completed study?	Dropped?	Reason	Dose adjustment
1	66	m	angina; prior coronary bypass; prior myocardial infarction	Propranolol 20 mg t.i.d.; warfarin sodium 5 mg daily; $KH_2 PO_4$	isosorbide dinitrate 10 mg three times daily; nitroglycerin sublingually as needed	no	yes	inadequate trial of dose adjustment; patient discontinued himself	1.0 mg q 6 h to 1.5 mg q 6 h then discontinued
2	39	m	angina; hypertension	propranolol 80 mg q 6 h; hydrochlorothiazide 50 mg daily	isosorbide dinitrate 5 mg q 6 h; nitroglycerin 0.4 mg as needed	no	yes	intolerable headaches during titration	dose titration only to 1.0 mg to 1.5 mg to 1.0 mg
3	53	m	angina	propranolol 40 mg four times daily	nitroglycerin 0.4 mg sublingually as needed	yes (March 6, 1981)	–	–	1.0 mg q 6 h to 1.5 mg q 6 h
4	68	m	angina; prior coronary bypass; prior myocardial infarction	propranolol 20 mg q.i.d.; triamterene + hydrochlorothiazide 1 tablet/day	isosorbide dinitrate 10 mg q.i.d.; isosorbide dinitrate 5 mg sublingually as needed	yes (February 23, 1981)	–	–	1.0 mg q 6 h
5	65	m	angina; prior coronary bypass; prior myocardial infarction	propranolol 80 mg b.i.d. to colchicine 0.6 mg daily; aspirin 2 tablets daily	nitroglycerin 0.6 mg sublingually as needed	yes (March 30, 1981)	–	–	1.5 mg q 6 h to 1.5 mg q 4 h to 2.0 mg q 4 h

Optimum outpatient dose	Optimum inpatient dose	Dissolution rate average	Side effects	Buccal mucosa	General response/ comments	Conti- nuation	Angina prior to study?	After study?
not applicable	not applicable	up to 6 h	none	no irritation	more angina with low-dose nitro-glycerin buccally than with isosorbide dinitrate; unable to continue with trial to reach optimum dose	not applicable	1–2/week	not applicable
not applicable	2.0 mg	not applicable	headache	–	dose titration only to 1.0 mg to 1.5 mg to 1.0 mg	not applicable	7/week	not applicable
1.5 mg q 6 h	1.0 mg	6 h	Occasional slight headache after 2nd daily dose; relieved with acetaminophen; no headache after 2 weeks	no irritation three times; injection three times	likes medication – infrequent episodes of angina with increased activity (unable to tolerate isosorbide dinitrate because of severe headache)	yes – 1.5 mg q 6 h; will return at monthly intervals	1–2/month	decreased with activity increase
1.0 mg q 6 h	1.25 mg (0.5–2.5 mg)	5–6 h (when working dissolved in 2 h)	none	injection once (2nd daily visit); no irritation for rest of study	good response; no angina; patient likes medication	yes – 1.0 mg q 6 h; will return at monthly intervals	?	decreased
2.0 mg q 4 h	2.5 mg	2–3 h	none	no irritation	feels definite improvement with nitro-glycerin buccally despite occasional exertional angina after heavy meals (not as severe with nitro-glycerin buccally)	yes – 2.0 mg q 4 h; will return at monthly intervals	15/week	occasional

Appendix (continued)

Patient No.	Age years	Sex	Diagnosis	Medication	Prior nitrates	Completed study?	Dropped?	Reason	Dose adjustment
6	56	m	angina	disopyramide 400 mg/day; propranolol 160 mg/day	0.4 mg nitroglycerin sublingually as needed	yes (March 31, 1981)	–	–	1.5 mg q 6 h to 1.0 mg q 6 h (lowered because of headache)
7	45	m	angina; arthritis	propranolol 40 mg q.i.d.; trilisate 500 mg q.i.d.; clidinium bromide + chlodiazepoxide as needed	0.3 mg nitroglycerin sublingually as needed	yes (March 31, 1981)	–	–	1.0 mg q 6 h to 1.0 mg q 4½ h to 1.0 mg q 4 h
8	65	m	angina; optic neuritis; controlled hypertension	propranolol 20 mg q.i.d.; anturane 200 mg q.i.d.; triamterene + hydrochlorothiazide 1 tablet/day	5.0 mg isosorbide dinitrate orally t.i.d.; 0.4 mg nitroglycerin sublingually as needed	yes (April 8, 1981)	–	–	1.0 mg q 6 h
9	51	m	angina;	nadolol 80 mg daily; lonazepam 0.5 mg as needed	isosorbide dinitrate 20 mg daily; 0.4 mg nitroglycerin sublingually as needed	yes (May 4, 1981)	–	–	1.0 mg q 6 h to 1.5 mg q 6 h to 2.0 mg q 6 h
10	53	f	angina; prior coronary bypass; prior thyroidectomy; hypothyroidism	metoprolol 300 mg q 6 h; valium 5 mg at night as needed; acetylsalicylic acid 600 mg as needed	isosorbide dinitrate 80 mg per os q 6 h; 0.3 mg nitroglycerin sublingually as needed	yes (April 7, 1981)	–	–	1.5 mg q 6 h to 1.5 mg q 4 h to 2.0 mg q 4 h to 2.5 mg q 3 h to 3.5 mg q 3 h to 5.0 mg q 3 h to 5.0 mg + isosorbide dinitrate 40 mg

Optimum outpatient dose	Optimum inpatient dose	Dissolution rate average	Side effects	Buccal mucosa	General response/ comments	Continuation	Angina prior to study?	After study?
1.0 mg q 6 h	1.0 mg	2.5–2.75 h	mild headache, relieved with acetaminophen	no irritation	somewhat improved; could tolerate (had to discontinue isosorbide dinitrate orally because of severe headaches)	no – little angina without nitroglycerin buccally	1/week	0
1.0 mg q 4 h	1.0 mg	4 h	slight throbbing type headache (mentioned once, relieved with aspirin)	injection three times; no irritation four times	likes medication; able to do more; less angina pain (had stopped isosorbide dinitrate because of headache and gastrointestinal symptoms)	yes – 1.0 mg q 4 h; will return at monthly intervals	10–15/week	decreased
1.0 mg q 6 h	1.0 mg	3–3.5 h	none	no irritation five times; injection two times	commented on improved appetite on two occasions and generally 'feeling better'	decided not to continue on medication, has very little angina	0	0
2.0 mg q 6 h	1.5 mg	6 h	mild headache, tolerable; less bothersome after taking medication for period of time	no irritation four times; slight injection twice; mild erythema once	prefers to remove tablet while eating; suggests schedule administering around meals; good response main benefit from morning dose	yes, will use as needed up to t.i.d. and return at monthly intervals	4–5/week	0
5.0 mg	1.5 mg	erratic 1–7 h	high dose headache and nausea	no irritation five times	inadequate response on 5.0 mg; still very symptomatic many days of week; no true rest pain; note: subsequent cardiac catheter, thallium: May 21, 1981	not applicable	?	?

Appendix (continued)

Patient No.	Age years	Sex	Diagnosis	Medication	Prior nitrates	Completed study?	Dropped?	Reason	Dose adjustment
11	54	m	exertional angina	hydrochlorothiazide 50 mg daily	pentaerythrol tetranitrate 1 tablet b.i.d.; 0.4 mg nitroglycerin sublingually as needed	yes (June 10, 1981)	–	–	1.0 mg q 6 h
12	66	m	increased angina; controlled hypertension; prior myocardial infarction; arthritis	propranolol 60 mg daily; furosemide 20 mg daily; aspirin 2 tablets; slow KCl	isosorbide dinitrate 5 mg sublingually four times daily	yes (June 8, 1981)	–	–	1.0 mg q 6 h
13	50	m	angina	propranolol 80 mg daily; aspirin 650 mg daily	isosorbide dinitrate 5 mg sublingually as needed	yes (June 17, 1981)	–	–	1.0 mg q 6 h to 1.5 mg q 6 h to 1.5 mg q 5 h to ↓ 1.0 mg q 5 h (headache) to 1.5 mg q 5 h
14	40	m	angina	hydrochlorothiazide 50 mg daily; propranolol 40 mg q.i.d.	isosorbide dinitrate 40 mg per os daily; 0.4 mg nitroglycerin sublingually as needed	yes (July 7, 1981)	–	–	1.5 mg q 6 h to 2.0 mg q 6 h
15	65	m	angina; adult-onset diabetes	chlorpropamide 750 mg daily; propranolol 240 mg daily	isosorbide dinitrate 120 mg daily	yes	–	–	1.0 mg q 6 h to 1.5 mg q 6 h to 2.0 mg q 6 h
16	55	m	angina	disopyramide 400 mg/day; propranolol 160 mg/day	isosorbide dinitrate 80 mg per os daily	yes (July 9, 1981)	–	–	1.5 mg q 6 h

Optimum outpatient dose	Optimum inpatient dose	Dissolution rate average	Side effects	Buccal mucosa	General response/ comments	Conti-nuation	Angina prior to study?	After study?
1.0 mg q 6 h	1.5 mg	3.5 h (when used at night, present in the morning)	mild headache, tolerable; decrease in severity after period of time	no irritation five times; injection two times	good response prevents angina during increased activity	yes, will use before increased activity and return monthly	occasional	0
1.0 mg q 6 h	1.5 mg	4–5 h	none	no irritation four times; injection three times	good response symptom free	yes, will continue with 1.0 mg t.i.d. and return monthly	4/week	0
1.5 mg q 5 h	1.0 mg	4–5 h	headache (bothersome on 1.5 mg, relieved with acetylsalicylic acid)	no irritation twice; injection four times	good response in prevention of angina on 1.5 mg; despite headache, patient chose to use 1.5 mg because of decreased angina	yes, continuing with 1.5 mg q 5 h, will return monthly	3–4/week	0
2.0 mg q 6 h	not applicable	left side 5–6 h right side 1.5–2.5 h	mild, infrequent headache	no irritation four times; injection three times	good response, feels it works better than nitroglycerin sublingually (cigarette smoker, drinker with poor dental hygiene)	yes, will continue with 2.0 mg as needed, will return monthly	?	0
2.0 mg q 6 h	not applicable	5–5.5 h	none	no irritation four times; injection twice; erythema once	good response; significant decrease in angina	yes, 2.0 mg q 6 h, monthly visits	5–6/week	2/week
1.5 mg q 6 h	not applicable	3–5 h	mild headache, none for the last 2 weeks of study	no irritation four times; injection three times	excellent response, no angina	yes, 1.5 mg t.i.d., monthly visits	?	0

Appendix (continued)

Patient No.	Age years	Sex	Diagnosis	Medication	Prior nitrates	Completed study?	Dropped?	Reason	Dose adjustment
17	45	m	angina; coronary artery disease; hyper-lipidemia	propranolol 80 mg daily	isosorbide dinitrate 2.5 mg sublingually as needed	yes (August 13, 1981)	–	–	1.0 mg q 6 h
18	60	m	angina; diabetes; osteo-arthritis; hyper-tension	methyldopa 1,000 mg daily; hydralazine HCl 20 mg daily; allopurinol 100 mg daily; vitamin B_{12} injection twice monthly	–	yes (August 17, 1981)	–	–	1.0 mg q 6 h to 1.5 mg q 6 h to 1.0 mg q 6 h (decreased because of headache on 1.5 mg)
19	60	m	angina; prior coronary bypass; prior myocardial infarction times four	digoxin 0.25 mg daily; propranolol 20 mg daily	isosorbide dinitrate 80 mg daily; 0.4 mg nitro-glycerin sublingually as needed	yes (October 28, 1981)	–	–	1.0 mg q 6 h to 1.5 mg q 6 h to 2.0 mg q 6 h to 3.0 mg q 6 h to 4.0 mg q 6 h to 5.0 mg q 6 h
20	54	f	angina; hyperten-sion	nitroglycerin propranolol (both occa-sionally)	nitroglycerin as needed	yes (October 28, 1981)	–	–	1.0 mg q 6 h to 1.5 mg q 6 h
21	54	m	angina; peptic ulcer history	propranolol 40 mg b.i.d.; cimetidine 300 mg at hour of sleep	isosorbide dinitrate 10 mg t.i.d.; nitroglycerin sublingually as needed	yes (November 20, 1981)	–	–	1.5 mg q 6 h to 2.0 mg q 6 h to 2.5 mg q 6 h
22	69	m	coronary artery disease; prior myocardial infarction times two	acetylsalicylic acid 300 mg daily	isosorbide dinitrate t.i.d. and 10 mg at night	yes (December 8, 1981)	–	–	1.0 mg q 6 h to 1.5 mg q 6 h to 2.0 mg q 6 h

Optimum outpatient dose	Optimum inpatient dose	Dissolution rate average	Side effects	Buccal mucosa	General response/ comments	Conti- nuation	Angina prior to study?	After study?
1.0 mg q 6 h	not applicable	6–7 h	slight to severe headache at beginning of study; no headache by end of study	no irritation three times; injection four times	likes psycho- logic effect of continued medication; wants to use 1.0 mg as needed and compare ef- fects with isosorbide dinitrate sublingually	yes, as needed, will return at monthly intervals	1/week	0
1.0 mg q 6 h	not applicable	5–7 h (1.0 mg longer lasting)	headache on 1.5 mg	no irritation four times; injection twice	gets no headache on 1.0 mg; was unable to tolerate other medi- cations due to headache; angina only when biking after medi- cation or uphill; therefore, ef- ficacy hard to determine	yes, as needed for biking to determine if it works; will return at monthly intervals	4/week	0
5.0 mg q 6 h	not applicable	7 h	none	no irritation six times; injection once	feels secure with tablet in place; able to increase ac- tivity with less angina	yes, will return weekly at first to evaluate the results of 5.0 mg	15–16/week	2/week
1.5 mg q 6 h	not applicable	6 h	headache (occipital); improved by end of study	no irritation six times; injection once	'I think it helped'; wants to con- tinue using it	yes, will return at monthly intervals	7/week	1–2/week
2.5 mg q 6 h	1.5 mg	4 h	headache, improved after 3rd day, gone by end of study	no irritation once; injection three times; slight erythema once	'this medicine has really helped to decrease the frequency and severity of angina attacks, espe- cially walk- ing uphill'	yes, will also use nitro- glycerin as needed and return at monthly intervals	21/week	0 (when tablet in place)
2.0 mg q 6 h	not applicable	6 h	none	no irritation five times; injection twice	good response; angina attacks decreased; 'I like it because I feel protected'	yes, 2.0 mg q 6 h, will return at 1- to 2-month intervals	5–6/week	1/week

Adv. Pharmacother., vol. 1, pp. 166–173 (Karger, Basel 1982)

Efficacy of Buccal Synchron Nitroglycerin in Patients with Angina pectoris

Edgar Lichstein, Alvin Greengart, Sanford Bolton, Gerald Hollander, Michael Sanders

Maimonides Medical Center, Downstate Medical Center, State University of New York, Brooklyn, N.Y., USA

This study was designed to evaluate the efficacy of a new controlled release form of nitroglycerin in the prevention of exercise induced angina using a well-established double-blind exercise protocol [1].

Exercise studies were performed on 16 patients. There were 15 males and 1 female with age ranging from 35 to 64 years. All patients had chronic stable exertional angina for at least 6 months prior to this study. The presence of coronary heart disease was documented by the presence of myocardial infarction in 15 and angiographic evidence of at least 50% obstruction in one or more coronary arteries in 14 patients.

Exertional angina was precipitated by bicycle exercise testing in all patients. All patients were evaluated on an outpatient basis. The initial evaluation included history, physical examination, electrocardiogram, chest X-ray, complete blood count, urinalysis and biochemical evaluation.

Propranolol, antiarrhythmic medication, diuretics and noncardiac medications were continued prior to and during this study. Digoxin therapy was discontinued at least 2 days prior to this study. Long-acting nitrates were gradually tapered prior to the study and discontinued at least 2 days prior to testing. The patients did not take any other long-acting nitrates throughout the duration of the study. During this time, the patients were instructed to use sublingual nitroglycerin for any episodes of exertional chest pain.

The dose of buccal Synchron nitroglycerin to be used in this study was determined by the following procedure. The pulse rate and blood pressure were measured prior to administration of buccal nitroglycerin until stable values were obtained. This was defined as less than a 10-mm Hg variation in systolic blood pressure and less than a ten beat per minute variation in heart rate. All patients were then given a 1-mg test dose of buccal nitroglycerin. The patient was instructed to insert the tablet in the upper buccal pouch between the cheek and the upper gum on either side. Heart rate, blood pressure and evaluation of the patient for symptoms such as headache and dizziness were recorded every 0.5 h for the first hour and then at hourly intervals for 5 h. A positive response was considered to be present if the dose produced a 10-mm Hg reduction in sitting systolic blood pressure and/or a 10 beat per minute increase in heart rate over baseline [2]. If a positive response was not noted, the patient was given a higher dose the following day. The patients received serial administration of higher doses (2.0, 2.5 and 5 mg) on succeeding days. All patients had a positive hemodynamic response to one of these doses of buccal Synchron nitroglycerin. This dose was then identified as the test dose for that patient. The time of dissolution of the tablet was also noted.

Practice bouts of exercise were performed on the bicycle ergometer on the second day at baseline prior to administration of a known placebo and then again at 1 and 3 h after its administration. On day 3, practice bouts of exercise were repeated at baseline and at 0.5, 1, 3 and 5 h after placebo. The exercise protocol for days 4 and 5 consisted of administration of double-blinded placebo and active buccal nitroglycerin of preselected dose. 14 of the 16 patients had a separate test dose of sublingual nitroglycerin 0.4 mg and all had a positive hemodynamic response as previously defined.

An individualized sequence of workload was selected for each patient so that in the absence of an active nitrate preparation, the onset of angina occurred within 3–5 min of exercise. Patients pedaled a Tunturi ergometer steadily at 50 revolutions per minute and workloads were increased by 20–25 W at 3-min intervals. Exercise was stopped and exercise duration recorded when the patient indicated the presence of angina or severe fatigue. The patients were continuously monitored using leads I, AVF and V5.

The dose of buccal nitroglycerin that produced a hemodynamic effect was used for the study and ranged from 1.0 to 5.0 mg with a mean of 3.1 mg. For patients on propranolol, the dose ranged from 1.0 to 5.0 mg with a mean of 3.2, and for those without propranolol the range was from 2.0 to 5.0 mg with a mean of 2.2.

The stability and reproducibility of this exercise protocol is shown by comparing the time of exercise duration at baseline on days 4 and 5 for both placebo and active medication. These times are shown in table I and are not significantly different.

The administration of buccal Synchron nitroglycerin produced a definite increase in duration of exercise when compared to placebo as is seen in the graph shown in figure 1. 13 of the 16 patients showed improvement. The maximum difference in exercise duration with buccal Synchron nitroglycerin was seen at 0.5 h. On medication, the mean duration of exercise was 239 s at baseline and increased to 334.7 s after buccal Synchron nitroglycerin. This is compared with a baseline duration of exercise of 236.6 s with placebo which remained exactly unchanged at 0.5 h. The difference is statistically significant ($p < 0.01$). An increased duration of exercise with buccal Synchron nitroglycerin as compared to placebo was noted and was also statistically significant at 1 h and at 3 h. This is summarized in table I. The average difference at 5 h was 0.5 min (13%). The result at 5 h just misses significance at the 5% level with a p value of approximately 0.06. The average difference at each time period (with the exception of 5 h) as well as the overall average difference for all hours together was statistically significant ($p < 0.01$). 10 patients maintained the tablet in their buccal pouch for 5 h or longer. The time of exercise duration for these 10 patients was analyzed separately. The result of this analysis is shown in figure 2. The duration of exercise for these 10 patients with buccal Synchron nitroglycerin was greater than placebo at all time periods tested including 5 h. These differences were all statistically significant. The last 9 patients received a higher dose (0.5 mg higher) and showed significant activity ($p < 0.05$) even at the fifth hour.

Buccal Synchron nitroglycerin did not produce prolonged severe headache in any patients. 6 patients noted a slight headache or heavy sensation. 2 patients felt flushed and 1 patient had slight dizziness. These sensations were not judged to be unpleasant by the patient and did not impair the patient's ability to function. Symptomatic orthostatic hypotension did not occur. The presence of the tablet was not annoying to the subjects and did not interfere with eating, drinking or conversation.

A second study now being concluded evaluates the safety and clinical usefulness of buccal Synchron nitroglycerin. 22 patients with coronary heart disease and angina pectoris have been studied to date. The patient characteristics and the methods of documenting their disease are similar to the previ-

Table I. Mean duration of exercise in 16 patients with angina pectoris at baseline (B) and at 0.5 hour, 1 hour, 3 hours, and 5 hours after administration of buccal nitroglycerin (drug) and placebo.

	Drug					Placebo				
	B	0.5 h	1 h	3 h	5 h	B	0.5 h	1 h	3 h	5 h
Average	239	334.7	334.4	313.8	294.1	236.6	236.6	259.7	246.3	256.6
± SD	46.2	87.4	70.8	57.4	61.6	35.1	41.8	54.6	43.8	66.3

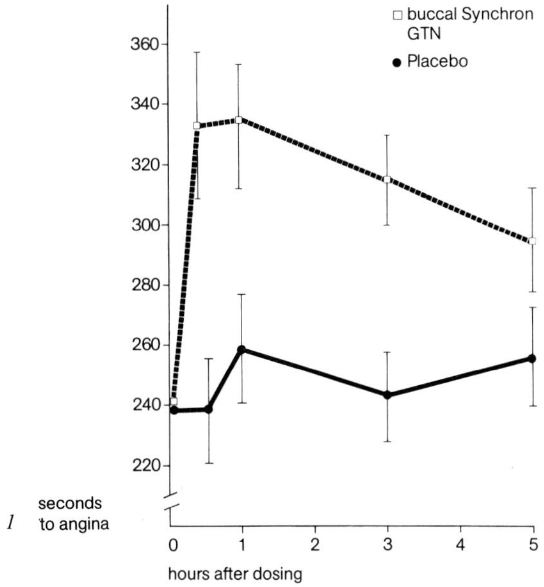

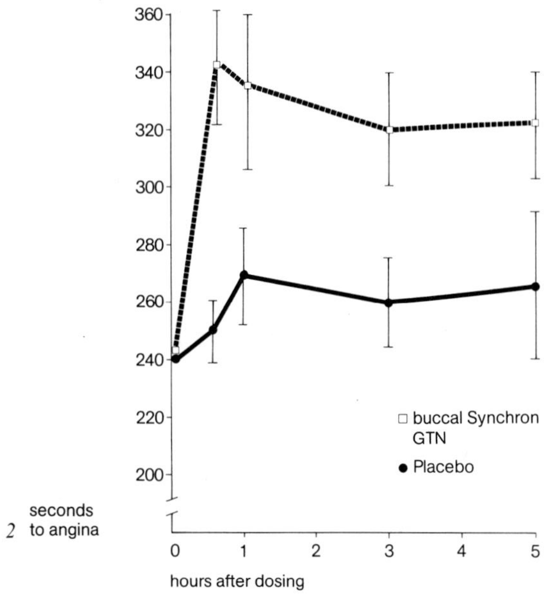

Fig. 1. Graph showing the difference in time to angina for all 16 patients.

Fig. 2. Graph illustrating time to angina for 10 patients in whom the buccal tablet was still present at 5 h.

ous study. During phase I, patients on long-acting nitrates were tapered off for 1 week and then kept off all nitrates for a second week. Phase II consisted of dose selection using response to blood pressure and heart rate as previously described. After dose selection, the patients were given buccal Synchron nitroglycerin of suitable dose and instructed to take the tablet three times daily. The individual dose for each patient, the time of hemodynamic response and the time to dissolution of the tablet are shown in table II. Phase III consisted of a 4-week period during which the patient continued to take buccal Synchron nitroglycerin and was seen once weekly for follow-up. The patient's course during this phase and comments are shown in table III. 8 of the last 10 patients who completed this study chose to continue on buccal Synchron nitroglycerin. The first 4 patients did not have this

Table II. Summary of open study of buccal synchron nitroglycerin (BNTG) indicating age, sex, dosage requirements, earliest onset of physiologic activity and the average dissolution time of BNTG in Phase III of the study

Patient No.	Sex	Age	Dose BNTG mg	Phase II time onset	Phase III average dissol. time
1	m	36	2.5 t.i.d.	3 min HA	4
2	m	59	1 t.i.d.	5 min HA ↓ BP	4
3	m	50	1.5 t.i.d.	5 min ↓ BP ↑ HR	3.5–4
4	m	57	1 t.i.d.	10 min ↓ BP ↑ HR	3–4
5	m	44	2 t.i.d. q 3 h	45 min ↓ BP	3–4
6	m	61	1.5 t.i.d.	3 min ↓ BP, ↑ HR	4.5–2
7	m	62	1/1.5 t.i.d.	3 min ↓ BP, ↑ HR	6
8	m	40	1/1.5	10 min ↓ BP	4–5
9	m	65	–	–	–
10	f	61	1 t.i.d.	5 min ↓ BP	6
11	m	52	1 t.i.d.	10 min ↓ BP	6–7
12	m	56	1 t.i.d.	5 min ↓ BP	6
13	m	52	1	5 min ↓ BP	–
14	m	41	1 t.i.d.	5 min ↓ BP	5
15	f	44	–	–	–
16	m	63	1 t.i.d.	7 min ↓ BP	1.5–2 was in phase II
17	m	56	–	–	–
18	m	57	1/1.5 t.i.d.	3 min ↓ BP	6
19	m	50	1 t.i.d.	5 min ↑ HR	6
20	f	46	1 t.i.d.	3 min ↓ BP	4
21	m	56	1 t.i.d.	1 min ↓ BP	6
22	m	49	1 t.i.d.	5 min ↓ BP	6

BNTG = buccal Synchron nitroglycerin; HA = headache; BP = blood pressure; HR = heart rate.

Table III. Course of disease and state of health of the patients during the 4-week BNTG treatment phase and comments for further treatment after end of study

Patient No.	Course and comments	Post phase III on BNTG
1	Less angina, headache as with other nitrates	Na
2	Less angina, mild headache	Na
3	Initial headache only; dissolution time longer at night (mouth dry)	Na
4	No angina, occasional dizziness, occasional burning from BNTG	Na
5	Less angina, initial headache only, faster dissolution of BNTG with liquids	yes
6	No angina	yes
7	Less angina, occasionally dislodged BNTG with dentures	yes
8	Less angina, tingling in mouth for the first 5 min, faster dissolution of BNTG with hot liquids	yes
9	Non cardiac disease interrupted study	–
10	No angina, mild headache, dry mouth probably related to hyperglycemia	yes
11	Occasional angina, slight headache	no
12	Occasionally swallowed BNTG which he promptly replaced; no angina	yes
13	Baseline BP 97/68 fell to 80/50 at 30 min; no symptoms but discontinued according to protocol	–
14	Headache from previous eighth nerve resection; prior headache from nitrates; headache with BNTG	–
15	Patient could not be withdrawn from nitrates; not continued in study	–
16	Less angina, mild headache; removes BNTG for eating	yes
17	Not continued in study because of scheduled bypass surgery	–
18	Less angina, headache phase II, none in phase III	yes
19	Headache requiring analgesic; this decreased during study	no
20	Headache requiring analgesic; BNTG lasted longer at night (8 h)	2 weeks in phase III
21	Less angina, mild headache, improving in phase III	1 week in phase III
22	Less angina	1 week in phase III

Na = not applicable, continuation of therapy not possible because FDA approval was not available; yes = after study was ended, the patient continued taking the drug; no = after study was ended, the patient discontinued.

option because FDA approval had not been granted. All patients noted an improvement in their symptoms with 36% having complete absence of angina pectoris. Mild headache occurred, as had occurred with the patient's other long-acting nitrates [3], and usually responded to analgesic therapy and frequently gradually subsided or disappeared. No patient developed irritation of the buccal mucosa.

We conclude that buccal Synchron nitroglycerin is an effective and well-tolerated controlled release nitrate which is well suited for clinical practice [3, 4]. Its beneficial characteristics include onset, prolonged duration of activity which may persist as long as 5 h, ability to easily titrate dose and predictable duration of action which can be judged by the patient with a minimum of side effects.

References

1 Redwood, D.R.; Rosing, D.R.; Goldstein, R.F.; Beiser, D.; Epstein, S.F.: Importance of the design of an exercise protocol in the evaluation of patient with angina pectoris. Circulation *43:* 618–628 (1971).

2 Reichek, N.: Long-acting nitrates in the treatment of angina pectoris. J. Am. med. Ass. *236:* 1399–1402 (1976).

3 Abrams, J.: Nitroglycerin and long-acting nitrates. New Engl. J. Med. *302:* 1234–1237 (1980).

4 Abrams, J.: Usefulness of long-acting nitrates in cardiovascular disease. Am. J. Med. *64:* 183–185 (1978).

E. Lichstein, MD, Maimonides Medical Center, Division of Cardiology,
State University of New York, 4802 Tenth Avenue, Brooklyn, NY 11219 (USA)

Discussion

Chairman: *W.-D. Bussmann*

Bussmann: Dr. *Lichstein,* did you also use the 5.0 mg tablets?

Lichstein: We used the 5.0 in a very small number of patients, but as the protocol dictated, it would only be used if a patient did not show a hemodynamic response to one of the lower doses – and that was unusual.

Bussmann: In 10% of the patients?

Lichstein: No, much smaller. Most patients responded to the lower dose.

Abrams: It's important to remember that although the protocol design is appropriate, that is looking for a blood pressure and heart rate response, it still is not clear, at least not to me, that the anti-anginal effect in a given individual is related to the increase in heart rate and/or the fall in blood pressure. And it is certainly conceivable that there will be patients who will respond to this buccal preparation, or others who may not show a clear-cut response hemodynamically and vice versa. I am sure there will be some patients who will get the blood pressure and heart rate change and in whom the anti-anginal action may not be seen. This is a truism about nitrates in general. I don't know how much we should focus on this in terms of a guideline for therapy.

Lichstein: Well, first of all it would help if we knew which effect of nitroglycerin alleviates angina, but if you believe in the other effect – the action on actually dilating the coronary arteries – from our experience in the cath lab, I think it's the same order of magnitude in about the same amount of time.

Reichek: I believe that the first part of what you said is unequivocally correct. That is, that one can demonstrate therapeutic effects without these heart rate and blood pressure effects. But there is now a substantial body of data accumulated by many different groups over more than a decade that would argue that if one identifies such a heart rate and blood pressure effect in a patient with exertional angina, one will see a therapeutic effect, and that this is quite consistent. Therefore, we have only used this as a threshold device to identify a dose which we think will be effective, and also to be able to match doses of different agents. Because, to my mind, one of the greatest problems in comparing any of these agents is to try to identify the same point in the dose-response curve for each agent in that individual. That's the way that we've used it. But I agree: I don't think it has anything to do directly with the therapeutic effect.

Adv. Pharmacother., vol.1, pp. 174–183 (Karger, Basel 1982)

Open Study of Safety and Tolerability of Nitroglycerin Buccal Controlled Release Tablet

E. Lichstein, A. Greengart, G. Hollander, M. Sanders, G. Cohen [1]
Maimonides Medical Center, Division of Cardiology, Brooklyn, N.Y., USA

Introduction

Sublingual administration of nitroglycerin (GTN) is used for the symptomatic relief of angina pectoris. Since it has a short duration of action, it is not an effective prophylactic agent. Attempts have been made to prolong the effect of GTN by altering its chemical configuration and method of administration. Our study was designed to evaluate the use of a small tablet containing GTN in an inert controlled release polymer which when placed in the buccal pouch introduces the GTN systemically (buccal Synchron nitroglycerin; BGTN). We have previously evaluated the efficacy of a single dose of BGTN in prolonging exercise tolerance in anginal patients in a double-blind study. We found a significant and prolonged increase in exercise tolerance for a 5-hour period with doses ranging from 1.0 to 5.0 mg. This study of BGTN was designed to evaluate the use of BGTN in the treatment of chronic angina pectoris. Our objectives were (1) to establish the safety and tolerability of BGTN; (2) to determine a useful repetitive dosing regimen, and (3) to determine the duration of changes in the physiologic responses of heart rate and blood pressure.

[1] The authors wish to acknowledge the assistance of Mrs. *Nancy Zimet*, RN, and Ms. *Danielle Harrison* for their technical assistance, Mrs. *Ellen Chimenti* and Mrs. *Shaye Komitau* for their secretarial assistance and manuscript preparation.

Materials and Methods

Population

26 patients started the study and 21 patients completed the protocol. 5 patients were excluded from the study for reasons which will be discussed below.

Patients between the ages 35 and 65 years with classic angina pectoris were eligible and volunteered for this study. The presence of coronary artery disease was documented by at least one of the following criteria: (1) selective coronary arteriography that showed 70% or greater narrowing of a major coronary artery or one or more of its primary branches (24 patients) and (2) electrocardiographic changes indicative of previous myocardial infarction or an ECG that showed ST-T wave or T wave changes plus a clinical history and serum changes indicative of a myocardial infarction (20 patients).

Patients had known angina pectoris of at least 3 months duration which had stabilized in severity and frequency. They had known relief of exertional angina with GTN sublingual. 8 patients with coronary artery bypass surgery had recurrence of angina pectoris and were at least 3 months after surgery. Patients were excluded if they had: (1) overt symptomatic congestive heart failure; (2) myocardial infarction within 3 months of the start of the observation period; (3) concomitant disease that may mimic the symptoms of angina pectoris, e.g., hiatus hernia, active ulcer disease, or costochondritis; (4) documented unstable or variant angina pectoris; (5) cerebrovascular disease, history of vascular headaches, uncontrolled hypertension and glaucoma; (6) anemia, thyrotoxicosis, and significant cardiac valvular disease; (7) intolerance to sublingual administration of GTN; (8) insulin-dependent diabetes.

18 patients were receiving propranolol in doses ranging from 40 to 480 mg daily. The mean dose of propranolol was 156 mg. 9 patients were receiving digoxin, 15 patients were receiving diuretics, and 4 patients received other antihypertensive medications. 2 patients were on long-acting oral hypoglycemics, 2 patients were receiving antiarrhythmics, and 2 patients were on thyroid replacement therapy. 20 patients were receiving other long-acting nitrate therapy prior to taking the BGTN tablet. These were tapered during phase I of the protocol.

Protocol

Phase I: Observation Period. The Observation period was 1 week for patients not taking long-acting nitrates, 1 week washout and 1 week observation period for patients taking long-acting nitrates. All patients were evaluated on an outpatient basis. The initial evaluation included a detailed history, physical examination, sitting and standing blood pressure in the same arm taken three times in each position, chest X-ray obtained within 3 months, complete blood count, biochemical evaluation and 12-lead electrocardiogram. The biochemical evaluation included: electrolytes, blood urea nitrogen, glucose, creatinine, alkaline phosphatase, serum glutamic oxaloacetic acid transaminase, serum glutamic pyruvic transaminase, bilirubin, calcium, phosphorus, albumin, globulin, total protein, and creatinine phosphokinase. Significant laboratory abnormalities were noted in several patients as follows: elevated white blood cell count – 2 patients (12,500–17,100), elevated blood glucose – 5 patients (160–449), elevated lactate dehydrogenase – 3 patients (251–357), elevated uric acid – 2 patients (8.5–10.6), elevated serum glutamic pyruvic transaminase – 1 patient (166), elevated calcium – 1 patient (11.8).

Patients not previously taking any long-acting nitrates were instructed to take GTN sublingual for acute episodes of angina pectoris only. The prophylactic use of GTN sublingual to prevent expected episodes of angina pectoris was prohibited. Patients who were taking long-acting nitrates were given a tapering schedule prescribed by the investigators over a 1-week period. If discontinuation of long-acting nitrates was successful, the patients were instructed to take GTN sublingual nitroglycerin only for acute episodes of angina. The patients were observed for 1 week off long-acting nitrates and then entered into the dose adjustment phase.

Phase II: Dosage and Adjustment Period. Phase II consisted of the dose selection trial and initial follow-up. Baseline resting heart rate and systolic and diastolic blood pressure were measured after the patient sat quietly for 10 min until stable values were obtained (variation less than 10 beats/min in heart rate and 10 mm Hg systolic blood pressure). The patients' buccal cavities were examined before BGTN was administered. Blood pressure and heart rate were obtained in the sitting position at baseline and 1, 3, 5, 7, 10, 15, 20, 30, 45, 60, 90, 120, 180, 240, 300, and 360 min after the BGTN tablet had been put into place. In addition, standing blood pressure and heart rate were obtained at 15, 30, 45, 60, 90, 120, 180, 240, 300, and 360 min.

The dosage was initially started with a single 1.0-mg BGTN tablet. The patients were instructed to place the tablet in one of the upper buccal pouches between the cheek and the gum, alternating right and left sides each time a tablet was taken. The optimal dose of the drug was defined as the minimum dose that produced a 10-beat/min increase in heart rate or 10 mm Hg decrease in systolic blood pressure in the sitting position without symptoms of orthostatic hypotension [1]. If the baseline systolic blood pressure was 100 mm Hg or less, a decrease in sitting and standing systolic pressure to 90 mm Hg without orthostatic symptoms defined the optimal dose of the drug. If the symptomatic orthostatic hypotension were to occur or the sitting systolic pressure were to decrease below 90 mm Hg, the BGTN tablet was to be discarded and the patient considered a dropout due to unavailability of a suitable dose.

If after 1 h of administration of 1 mg BGTN there was no significant change in heart rate or blood pressure as previously defined, the tablet was removed, and the patient rested for 2 h. Then a 1.5-mg BGTN tablet was administered and the protocol as defined previously was repeated. If after 1 h no significant physiologic effect was noted, another 2-hour rest period was taken. A 2.0-mg tablet was then administered. If no response as defined above was seen within 1 h after administration, the tablet was removed and the patient instructed to return on the following day for further titration with 2.5-mg and 5.0-mg tablets until an effective dose was defined. The patients were instructed to administer a BGTN tablet upon arising and then at 6-hour intervals for a total daily dose of 3 BGTN tablets.

The patient was then seen in follow-up daily for the first 3 days at 1 h after administration of the second dose with sitting and standing blood pressure and heart rate recorded. The buccal mucosa was also examined at this time.

Patients not successfully titrated did not enter the third phase of the study, but were discontinued and placed on conventional therapy.

Phase III: Follow-Up. Patients successfully completing phase II were continued at their optimal dosage on a Q 6 H × 3 daily schedule or as adjusted for 4 additional weeks. The patients were seen at weekly intervals to report any adverse effects. At each weekly visit sitting and standing blood pressure and heart rate were measured 1 h after the second dose. The patients were questioned concerning the palatability and acceptability of usage of the BGTN tablet and how long the tablet remained in the mouth. The buccal cavities were examined at each visit to observe for areas of irritation. The patients were asked about the usage of GTN sublingual for management of acute episodes of angina pectoris. Upon completion of phase III the patients had a follow-up laboratory examination including complete blood count and biochemical profile and follow-up electrocardiogram.

Results

26 patients entered into the protocol (table I). 3 patients entered phase I only. 2 of these 3 patients developed symptoms during the period when their nitrates were being tapered and could not continue in the protocol. 1 patient decided not to continue after phase I because of the scheduling of his coronary artery bypass surgery. 23 patients entered phase II. 1 patient (No. 13) developed a transient decrease in blood pressure from baseline of 97/68 to 80/50 30 min after administration of a 1-mg BGTN tablet. Although he was asymptomatic and had no orthostatic hypotension at this time, the protocol called for discontinuation from the study. Of the remaining 22 patients, 21 patients completed phase III. 1 patient (No. 14) had to be taken off the study in phase III because of severe unilateral occipital headache which did not respond to analgesic therapy. This patient had a previous 8th cranial nerve resection which produces a vestibulospinal reflex characterized by unilateral occipital pain. According to the patient's otolaryngologist this reflex was exaggerated by the use of GTN.

The dose of BGTN required to produce the previously defined hemodynamic effect ranged from 1.0 to 2.5 mg with a mean dose of 1.15 mg.

19 of 23 patients in phase II had an initial hemodynamic response to the 1-mg BGTN dose. The duration of activity as measured by the physiologic responses of heart rate and blood pressure in general paralleled the presence of the BGTN tablet in the buccal pouch. In 8 out of 22 patients, in whom the tablet remained for 6 h, the activity was demonstrated for at least 6 h after which measurements were stopped. In 5 of 22 patients, in whom the tablet dissolved before the 6th h, activity was demonstrated for 90 min to 2 h (mean 1.8 h) after the tablet was dissolved. In 2 of the 22 patients the physiologic activity returned to baseline before the tablet dissolved, 1 of whom subsequently required a higher dose for clinical reasons to control his angina. The peak activity of BGTN as measured by the maximum change in physiologic response occurred for the 23 patients in phase II between 5 and 120 min (mean 34 min) following drug administration. Of the 21 patients who completed phase III, 18 remained on the same dose and dosing schedule throughout the study, 2 patients (No. 8, 18) were given a higher dose to better control

Table I. Summary of clinical status, dose requirements and average dissolution time of BGTN, course of study and indication if patient chose to continue using BGTN after completion of study

Patient No.	Sex	Age years	Diagnosis	Recent prior nitrates	Other medication	BGTN mg	Phase III average dissolution time, h	After phase III on BGTN	Course and comments
1	m	36	ASHD, ANGIO after MI after CABG chronic hepatitis	none, because of headache	digoxin lasix prazosin	2.5 TID	4	not available	less angina, but disliked headache as he had with other long-acting nitrates; required analgesics
2	m	59	ASHD after MI	–	propranolol	1 TID	4	not available	less angina, mild headache
3	m	50	ASHD, ANGIO diabetes hypertension	isordil per os	propranolol diabinese hydrodiuril KCl	1.5 TID	3.5–4	not available	no angina, occasional dizziness and headache, burning from tablet for a few minutes
4	m	57	ASHD, ANGIO after MI after CABG	isordil per os	propranolol digoxin lasix, valium	1 TID	3–4	not available	no angina, occasional dizziness and headache, burning from tablet for a few minutes
5	m	44	ASHD, ANGIO after CABG	isordil sublingual	propranolol	2 TID	3–4	yes, requiring increased frequency	less angina and of decreased intensity; headache disappeared during phase III; after phase III requires four times 3-h dose because of nonischemic pain in surgical scar immediately following dissolution
6	m	61	ASHD, ANGIO after MI after CABG hypertension	nitrobid capsule nitro ointment	aldomet dyazide digoxin	1.5 TID	4.5	yes	on 2 mg had dizziness without orthostatic blood pressure change in phase II, no angina; average dissolution time faster following phase III (2 h)
7	m	62	ASHD, ANGIO after MI	ISDN per os	propranolol digoxin lasix KCl	1 TID	6	yes, requiring increased dose	significant decrease in angina; mild headache; occasionally dislodged BGTN with dentures; stress at home produced angina in follow-up after study, relieved by dose increase to 1.5 TID
8	m	40	ASHD, ANGIO after MI	nitrospan capsules	propranolol	1/1.5 TID	4.5	yes, 1 month only	markedly reduced angina, more active; dose increased in phase III to 1.5 mg for better angina control
9	m	65	ASHD, ANGIO after MI after CABG	isordil per os nitro ointment	propranolol lasix digoxin	–	–	–	study interrupted when noncardiac disease required hospitalization as patient was tapered off other nitrates
10	f	61	ASHD, ANGIO after MI after CABG diabetes	nitrobid capsules	digoxin lasix diabinese tolinase	1 TID	6	yes, 1 month only	no angina; mild headache, occasional analgesics; dry mouth, probably related to marked hyperglycemia; after study follow-up discontinued because of hospitalization
11	m	52	ASHD, after MI	nitrobid capsules sorbitrate	propranolol pronestyl	1 TID	6–7	no	occasional angina; slight headache; preferred BGTN to other nitrates, but declined to continue
12	m	56	ASHD, ANGIO after MI	ISDN per os	propranolol hydrodiuril	1 TID	6	yes	no angina; felt 'medication was great'; occasionally swallowed tablet
13	m	52	ASHD, ANGIO after MI	isordil per os nitro ointment	propranolol	1[1]	–	–	[1] phase II only; baseline blood pressure 97/64 fell to 80/50 at 30 min; no symptoms or orthostatic blood pressure change, but discontinued according to protocol

Table I (continued)

Patient No.	Sex	Age years	Diagnosis	Recent prior nitrates	Other medication	BGTN mg	Phase III average dissolution time, h	After Phase III on BGTN	Course and comments
14	m	41	ASHD, ANGIO after CABG hypertension	none, because of headache	propranolol hygroton serax	1 TID	5	did not complete phase III	angina improved, but significant unilateral occipital headache due to reflex from previous eighth nerve resection caused withdrawal in phase III; had previous headache from nitrates
15	f	44	ASHD, ANGIO diabetes hypertension	nitrobid capsules	propranolol esidrix	–	–	–	patient could not be withdrawn from nitrates and not continued in study
16	m	63	ASHD, ANGIO after MI	nitrobid per os	propranolol	1 TID	1.5–2	yes, but less than 1 month	angina much improved; mild headache; removed tablet for eating
17	m	56	ASHD, ANGIO after MI	nitrobid capsules nitro ointment	quinaglute valium, synthroid lanoxin	–	–	–	not continued in study after phase I because of scheduled coronary artery bypass surgery
18	m	57	ASHD, ANGIO hypertension	ISDN per os	methyldopa propranolol hydrodiuril	1/1.5 TID	6	yes	less angina; which resolved completely after dose was increased to 1.5 mg in phase III; headache in phase II, none in phase III
19	m	50	ASHD, ANGIO after MI	isordil 2.5 mg per os	propranolol	1 TID	6	no	no angina; had headache requiring analgesics, decreasing in severity during study; this, however, was bothersome; did not use higher dose isordil because of headache also
20	f	46	ASHD, ANGIO after MI hypertension	nitrobid capsules	inderide propranolol	1 TID	4	yes, but discontinued by private physician	angina improved and angina free at end of phase III; headache requiring analgesics early in phase III which disappeared during study
21	m	56	ASHD, ANGIO angina	nitrobid capsules	propranolol	1 TID	6	yes	angina improved; mild headache which improved in phase III; after the study had dizziness, and dose decreased to ½ tablets TID
22	m	49	ASHD, ANGIO after MI after CABG	–	persantin ASA, halfon	1 TID	6	yes	angina significantly improved; rare headache
23	f	55	ASHD, ANGIO after MI hypertension	–	propranolol hydrodiuril synthroid	1 TID	6	yes	angina significantly improved, with increase in activity; initial headache requiring analgesic which disappeared in phase III
24	m	47	ASHD, ANGIO after MI	–	–	1 TID/ QID	4	yes	during phase III, began to have angina after dissolution; dosage frequency increased to QID with complete relief
25	f	57	ASHD, ANGIO after MI hypertension	ISDN per os	digoxin lasix aldomet	1 TID	6	yes	marked improvement in angina with only rare episodes
26	m	58	ASHD, ANGIO after MI	ISDN per os	digoxin propranolol hydrodiuril	1 TIS	5	yes	angina markedly improved; headache early in phase III, relieved by coffee and resolved

ASHD = Atherosclerotic heart disease; ANGIO = coronary angiography; MI = myocardial infarction; CABG = coronary artery bypass graft surgery; TID = three times a day; ISDN = isosorbide dinitrate; QID = four times a day.

their anginal symptoms and 1 patient (No. 24) required an increased dosing frequency from three times to four times a day for symptom control.

After patient No. 4 FDA approval of these dosage forms was received, and the volunteers were offered the opportunity to continue using BGTN for chronic treatment of their angina pectoris.

17 patients were, therefore, offered continued use of BGTN after completion of the study protocol and 15 patients accepted.

2 patients chose not to continue (No. 11 for unexplained reasons; No. 19 because of headache symptoms). Of the 15 patients who continued, 4 patients continued for less than 1 month (No. 8 could not return for follow-up visit, No. 10 was hospitalized elsewhere for control of diabetes, No. 16 developed dizziness at times and tablet discontinued by private physician, No. 20 discontinued by private physician because of lack of experience with this drug).

In the follow-up phase, 1 patient (No. 7) required an increased dose from 1.0 to 1.5 mg to control anginal symptoms, and another patient (No. 5) required increased frequency of dosing because of the development of pain in his thoracotomy scar immediately after dissolution of the tablet (dosing frequency increased to Q3H). This pain was shown to be nonischemic by ECG monitoring during pain. Patient No. 21 required decreasing dose of BGTN to half of the scored 1-mg tablet because of episodic dizziness during an upper respiratory infection. Of the 21 patients who completed phase III, 33% (7/21) reported no angina during this study and 67% (14/21) reported a significant improvement in their angina.

No patient developed irritation of the buccal mucosa. 16 of the 21 patients who completed phase III had complaints of headache during the study. In 6 patients the headache disappeared during the course of this study, and in 8 patients the headache was characterized as mild, brief or intermittent. 2 patients (No. 1, 19) felt the headache to be significant und requiring frequent analgesic therapy. As previously noted, 1 patient (No. 14) was discontinued during phase III because of unilateral occipital headache. 1 patient (No. 4) had mild occasional dizziness. 50% of the patients had a tingling or burning sensation for a few minutes after insertion of the tablet. No patient experienced significant or prolonged local discomfort. 1 patient complained of a 'chalky' taste (No. 1), and 1 patient (No. 22) noted a 'peppermint' taste.

The average time for dissolution of the tablet was noted for the 21 patients in phase III. This varied from 1.75 h to as long as 6.5 h while awake. (If patients gave a range of times such as 6–7 h, this time was recorded as 6.5 h for statistical purposes.) The mean dissolution time in the patients was 4.7 h.

6 patients had some interference from the buccal tablet with eating. In order to maintain a three times a day dosing schedule, some patients removed the tablet for meals and a few scheduled their meals at appropriate intervals, so that the tablet was not present for their meals. Several patients had dentures which only occasionally dislodged the tablet, and some felt dentures protected the tablet against easy dissolution. For some patients, dissolution was noted to occur more rapidly when liquids, especially warm liquids, were ingested. A few patients reported the tablet remaining in the buccal pouch throughout the night if they had fallen asleep with the BGTN tablet still undissolved.

In the follow-up laboratory examination, no patient developed new electrocardiographic abnormalities. 1 patient (No. 4) had a decrease in serum calcium to 7.9 mg from baseline of 9.5 mg. 1 patient (No. 14) had slight increase in serum glutamic oxaloacetic acid transaminase several weeks after discontinuing BGTN therapy. This patient subsequently developed significant gallbladder disease requiring surgery. No other laboratory abnormalities were noted to occur during the study period.

Discussion

Desirable characteristics of long-acting nitrates that would be clinically useful for treatment of angina pectoris include rapid onset, prolonged duration, potent effect, easy dose titration and minimum or absence of side-effects. Our protocol selected a dose of BGTN with defined hemodynamic effect at 1 h after administration. The duration of the physiologic effect, in general, paralleled the presence of the undissolved BGTN tablet. This duration of action is easily judged by the patient who can easily check for the presence of the BGTN tablet in his buccal pouch.

The duration of the tablet in the buccal pouch before total dissolution varied from 1.75 to 6.5 h. The duration was longer in some patients who fell asleep with the BGTN tablet still in place. The mean dissolution time was 4.7 h. This dissolution time makes the BGTN preparation suitable for a three times a day or four times a day dosage schedule. For patients who find that dissolution of the tablet occurs more rapidly, it is possible to check for its presence and replace it as frequently as necessary. In most patients, the physiologic effects were at least as long as or sometimes longer than its physical presence. The physical presence of the tablet, however, may be reassuring to patients who feel they have prophylaxis against angina during that time.

The potent effect of the BGTN tablet is demonstrated by the significant reduction or elimination of angina pectoris in all the patients who completed phase III. 7 patients reported no angina during phase III, and 14 patients were significantly improved. 3 patients had dosage adjustment during phase III to improve their angina and 2 of these became angina free. In the other patients who experienced occasional episodes of angina, chronic therapy with a higher dose was not clinically required, although we can speculate that intermittent use of BGTN or increase in dosage may have provided them acute protection against expected angina-producing activity. This, however, was not offered to the patients.

16 of the 21 patients who completed phase III had been on other long-acting nitrates prior to using BGTN, and all noted improvement in their anginal syndrome when on the buccal tablet as compared to their previous nitrate preparations.

It is thought that the improvement in these patients was due to the continuous systemic release of active GTN by administration through the buccal route.

The side-effects of BGTN were similar to the commonly noted side-effects of other long-acting nitrates [2, 3]. Headache was the most common and was present at some time in 16 of 21 patients completing the study protocol. In 6 patients headache disappeared during phase II. In 8 patients, headache was only mild and intermittent. Only 2 of the 21 patients felt the headache to be significant requiring frequent analgesic therapy. Both patients had headache with other forms of long-acting nitrates. 1 additional patient had a predisposing cause to headache (ear surgery). This parallels the experience with other forms of nitrates where relief from headache can be expected with chronic use [2]. 1 patient had occasional dizziness, and 1 patient had a systolic blood pressure below 90 mm Hg, although he was asymptomatic. Occasional tingling of the buccal mucosa or burning sensation was noted initially and usually disappeared within a few minutes. This was not considered significant by any of the patients.

No patient had any irritation of the buccal mucosa. No patient had any difficulty in speaking or drinking. 2 patients noted a different taste, 1 'chalky' and 1 'peppermint'. Several patients noted that the tablet would shift its position or be swallowed with eating, but this was managed by removing the tablet and replacing it after eating or by scheduling meals at appropriate intervals so that the BGTN tablet was not present. This was done so that the three times a day dosage schedule according to the protocol could be maintained. In clinical practice, however, the patients can insert a new tablet in case their usual eating habits caused accidental swallowing of the tablet, so that regular eating and drinking habits do not have to be disturbed.

The majority of the patients had a hemodynamic response to the 1-mg BGTN tablet.

Three patients had their dose increased from 1 mg to 1.5 mg either in phase III or in the post-study phase. 1 patient required decreased dosage from 1 mg in the post-study phase. None of the patients in whom the dose was increased had any adverse reactions from the increased dose. The mean time for peak hemodynamic effect was slightly over 30 min. This may be useful to advise patients about the time course of any side-effect.

The study suggests that patients to be started on buccal GTN should receive an initial dose of 1 mg with increasing dosage given if clinical symptoms require higher dosage.

Conclusion

We conclude that BGTN is a highly effective long-acting nitrate preparation. Its beneficial characteristics include rapid onset and prolonged duration of activity which can be judged by the patient. It is very effective in controlling symptoms of angina pectoris. The initial starting dose of 1.0 mg did not produce symptomatic hypotension in any patient. Adverse effects of BGTN therapy are similar to the other long-acting nitrate preparations available. These include headache and rare episodes of dizziness. A few patients had interference with eating requiring occasional removal and/or replacement of the tablet. The route of administration in the buccal cavity was acceptable to the majority of patients.

References

1 Reichek, N.: Long-acting nitrates in the treatment of angina pectoris. J. Am. med Ass. *236:* 1399–1402 (1976).

2 Abrams, J.: Nitroglycerin and long-acting nitrates. New Engl. J. Med. *302:* 1234–1237 (1980).

3 Abrams, J.: Usefulness of long-acting nitrates in cardiovascular disease. Am. J. Med. *64:* 183–185 (1978).

E. Lichstein, MD, Maimonides Medical Center, Division of Cardiology,
State University of New York, 4802 Tenth Avenue, Brooklyn, NY 11219 (USA)

Adv. Pharmacother., vol.1, pp. 184–193 (Karger, Basel 1982)

Hemodynamic Effects of Oral Synchron Nitroglycerin in Comparison to Slow-Release Isosorbide Dinitrate

H.-U. Lehmann, E. Witt, P. Traue, H. Hochrein

III. Medizinische Klinik, Rudolf-Virchow-Krankenhaus, Berlin

Introduction

The clinical effects of nitroglycerin are essentially due to its peripheral actions in the large veins of the capacitive system. Vasodilatation leads to increased venous pooling with a decrease in right cardiac influx pressure. This is accompanied by what is often a substantial reduction in arterial resistance with a subsequent drop in systemic arterial pressure. Both mechanisms diminish the preload and afterload of the heart and thereby also the cardiac filling volume and the related ventricular wall tension, which is one of the significant myocardial O_2 determinants [2, 5, 7, 8, 12]. In contrast, the direct coronary vasodilative properties of nitroglycerin are of only relatively minor clinical significance. Reduction in myocardial O_2 demand and relief of heart performance are pharmacologic effects which can be used therapeutically for the management of angina pectoris and myocardial failure. However, this drug seems to be unsuitable for prophylaxis and long-term treatment of coronary heart diseases as it has a very short action of at most 20–40 min [9, 11, 12] due to its rapid inactivation during the liver passage [8]. For this indication long-acting nitrates were developed, e.g. isosorbide dinitrate (ISDN), trolnitrate, or pentaerthrityl tetranitrate, and also sustained release forms of nitroglycerin which can have prolonged effects as a result of a controlled release of the active substance [1, 3, 6, 10, 13]. Recently, Synchron nitroglycerin has been developed with the aim of sustaining its effects for up to 8 h [4]. For a more objective assessment of these findings, which are still controversial at the present time, hemodynamic tests on the effectiveness of cellulose-retarded nitroglycerin were carried out using ISDN as comparative therapeutic standard.

Patients and Methods

The study was designed as a randomized double-blind test including 40 patients. The method made provision for an intermediate analysis of the first 20 test results to decide whether there were sufficient arguments to justify a continuation of the study.

The result of this intermediate evaluation is the subject of our presentation. 20 patients were examined – 8 women and 12 men with an average age of 60.6 ± 10.1 years (between 40 and 72 years of age). All patients were suffering from coronary heart disease with clinically overt angina pectoris, where cardiac catheterization was indicated for diagnostic or therapeutic reasons. At the time of the study and during the preceding 3 days of the patients received any cardiac medication, neither nitrates nor beta-adrenoceptor blockers. Further basic therapy remained unchanged. Each patient had been previously informed as to the purpose and aim of the examination and had given his consent to the procedure.

Right cardiac catheterization was carried out by means of a three-lumenal Swan-Ganz thermodilution catheter with zero adjustment in the center of the thorax. Cardiac output was determined according to the thermodilution method (cardiac output computer, Edwards Laboratories, Mass., USA) and systemic arterial pressure was measured noninvasively.

The following circulation parameters were used for the evaluation: Right atrial pressure (RAP), pulmonary artery pressure (PAP), pulmonary artery wedge pressure (PCP), heart rate (HR), cardiac output (HMV), cardiac index (CI), stroke volume and stroke volume index (LVSWI) and total peripheral vascular resistance (TPR). Additional test parameters were: plasma level of nitroglycerin, subjective complaints, angina pectoris frequency.

The test program carried out for each patient consisted of a preliminary phase and an 8-hour control phase following administration of the drug. The test drug was administered according to a randomized double-blind protocol. The test drug contained either: 10 mg oral Synchron nitroglycerin (group I), 20 mg oral Synchron nitroglycerin (group II), 40 mg ISDN in sustained release formulation (group III), or placebo (group IV). The measurements were recorded at hourly intervals, beginning with phase 0 (preliminary phase) and finishing at the end of the 8th control hour. In addition, altogether 3 exercise testings were performed for each patient, one in the preliminary phase, a second after 4 h and the last after 8 h. The individual exercise tolerance determined in the preliminary phase (watts × minutes/product) was kept constant in control examinations.

Allocation to the groups was randomized and resulted in the following distribution: group I (10 mg cellulose-retarded nitroglycerin) consisted of 3 patients, group II (20 mg cellulose-retarded nitroglycerin) of 5, group III (40 mg isosorbide dinitrate in sustained release form) of 6, and group IV (placebo) also of 6 patients. The one-way analysis of variance was used for the calculations of significance.

Results

Oral Synchron Nitroglycerin. In the control phase both group I with 10 mg and group II with 20 mg cellulose-retarded nitroglycerin showed a significant and comparable, non-dosage-related drop in PAP and PCP whose maximum was reached after 1 h. The effect of the agent could be reliably

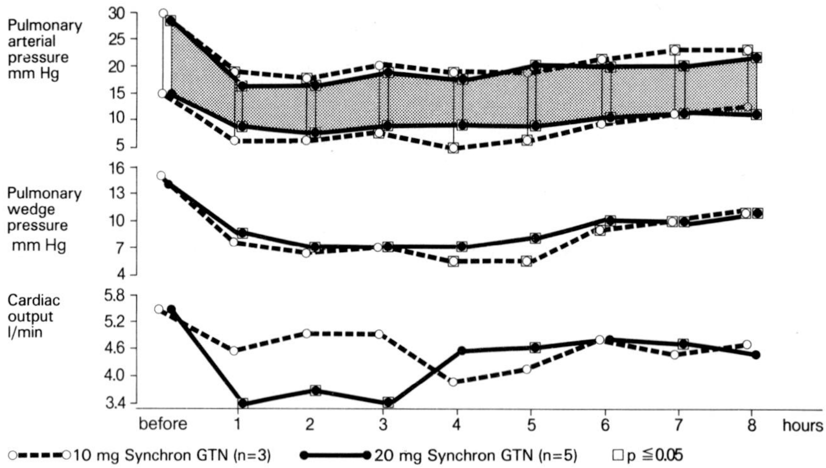

Fig. 1. Influence of Synchron GTN on the pressure values in the pulmonary circulation and on the cardiac output.

detected until the 6th hour. Even after 8 h the values were distinctly lower than the baseline values (fig. 1). This correlated with a simultaneous significant decrease in right atrial pressure. 10 mg cellulose-retarded nitroglycerin led to a slight reduction in cardiac output and SV; in the case of 20 mg this reduction was more pronounced and lasted until the 3rd control hour. In both groups the left ventricular stroke work index decreased significantly until the 8th hour. Heart rate tended to increase, particularly in group I, whereas systemic arterial pressure tended to decrease irrespective of group allocation.

ISDN in Sustained Release Form. In group III, which was treated with 40 mg ISDN, PAP, PCP, RAP, cardiac output, and SV basically reacted in the same manner (fig. 2). Here, too, the maximum effect was reached after the first hour, could reliably be identified until the 6th hour and slowly diminished between then and the 8th hour. The left ventricular stroke work index showed a significant decrease up to the 7th hour. This group differed from those receiving oral Synchron nitroglycerin in respect of heart rate which did not increase. A significant drop in systemic arterial pressure lasted until the 4th hour.

Placebo. Group IV, without pharmacologic treatment, also showed a significant drop in pulmonary pressure values although in comparison to groups I–III the differences were much less pronounced. Systemic arterial

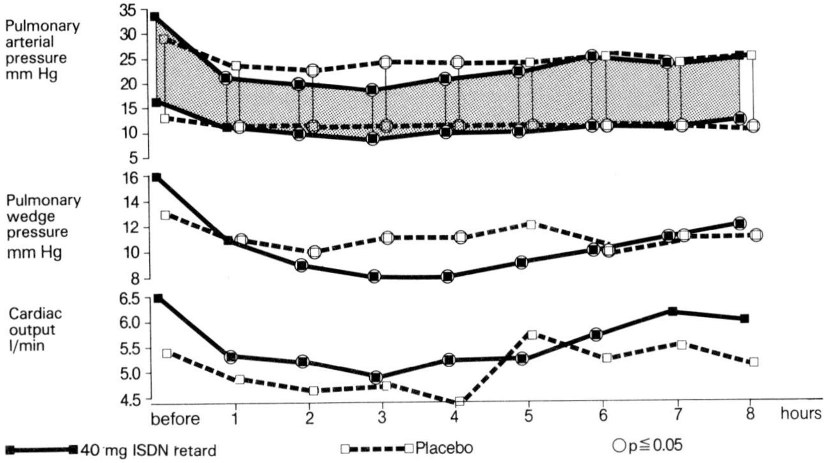

Fig. 2. Pulmonary arterial pressure, mean pulmonary wedge pressure and cardiac output following administration of ISDN retard and placebo.

pressure tended to decrease as well, but average cardiac output and stroke volume remained unchanged. The comparison with the drug groups shows the major difference to be a significant and more marked reduction in heart rate.

Comparison of Hemodynamic Action. A direct group comparison concerning the extent and duration of hemodynamic effects can be obtained by determining the differences between the baseline value and respective control measurements. ISDN and also oral Synchron nitroglycerin in both dosage forms produced a prolonged drop in pulmonary artery and pulmonary artery wedge pressure until the 6th hour, with the extent of these changes not varying from group to group (fig. 3, 4). ISDN and the higher dosage of oral Synchron nitroglycerin (20 mg) led to a reduced 3-hour cardiac output taken to be a result of the agents' effectiveness (fig. 5). In contrast, hemodynamic differences still persisting in the 7th and 8th hours cannot be reliably interpreted as drug effects alone since it is evident that considerable changes in hemodynamic reaction can be induced by resting for several hours as is shown by the result in the placebo group.

Exercise Stress Testing. Identical exercise conditions after the two oral Synchron nitroglycerin dosage forms and ISDN led to significant decreases in pulmonary artery and pulmonary artery wedge pressure in the 4th hour

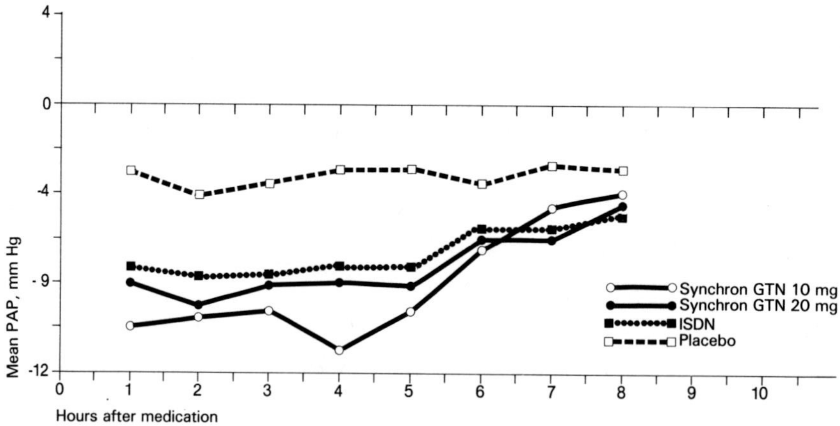

Fig. 3. Differences of mean pulmonary arterial pressure to initial value prior to medication (measuring at rest).

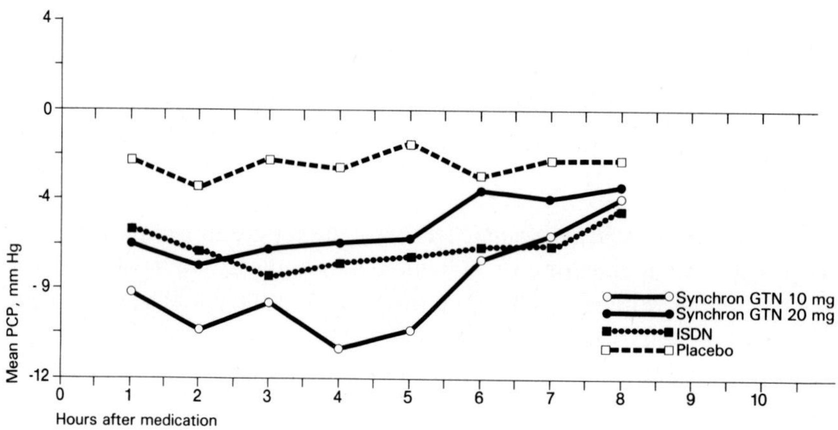

Fig. 4. Differences of mean pulmonary wedge pressure to initial value prior to medication (measuring at rest).

post application, however, without any quantitative differences. In contrast, cardiac output showed no specific changes (fig. 6). After 8 h no remaining effects of the drug could be detected.

Plasma Concentration of Nitroglycerin. Plasma concentration values of nitroglycerin varied between 0.2 ng/ml and excessively high concentrations exceeding 5 ng/ml in groups I and II. There was no correlation between dos-

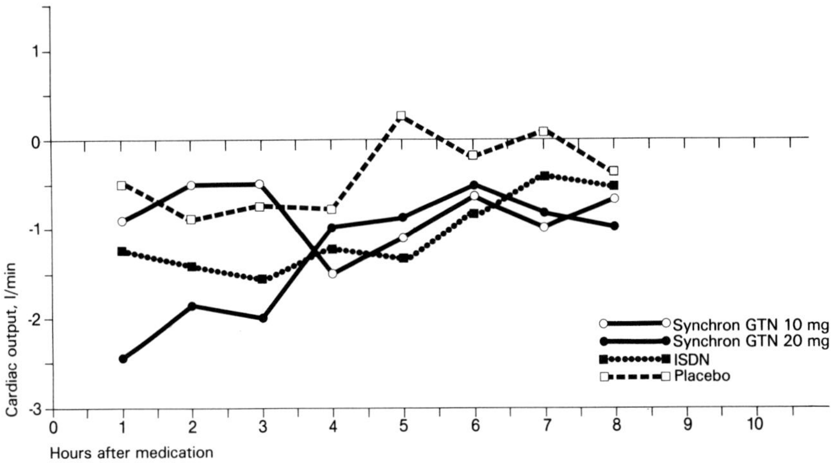

Fig. 5. Differences of cardiac output to initial value prior to medication (measuring at rest).

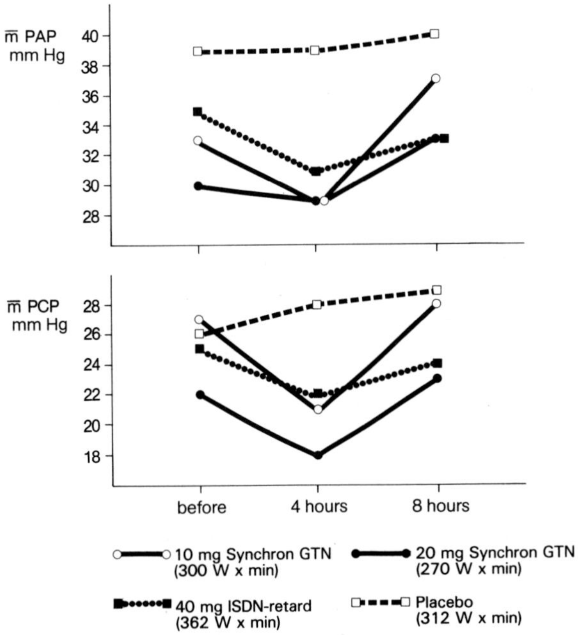

Fig. 6. Influence of Synchron GTN, ISDN retard and placebo on the pressure values in the pulmonary circulation under ergometric load.

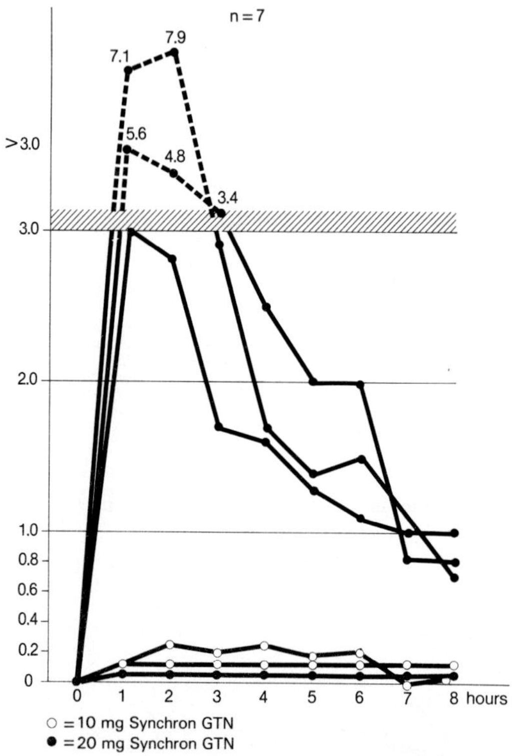

Fig. 7. GTN serum level during oral GTN treatment (ng/ml).

age and plasma concentration. Assays in altogether 5 patients from group II, who had received 20 mg oral Synchron nitroglycerin each, showed that 2 patients had ineffective, low plasma concentrations of less than 0.2 ng/ml while the other 3 had excessively high values which in 1 case went up to 7.9 ng/ml. In these 3 patients the plasma concentration after 8 h was still around 0.8 ng/ml (fig. 7).

The blood plasma of 2 patients in group I, who had received only 10 mg oral Synchron nitroglycerin, showed low concentration values between 0.2 and 0.4 ng/ml. No convincing correlation could be established between plasma concentration and hemodynamic effects.

Determination of nitroglycerin plasma concentration in the ISDN and placebo groups, which were done blindly, gave a false positive result in 1 out of 3 cases.

Side Effects. Migraine-like headaches were experienced in 2 cases of oral Synchron treatment and in 1 with ISDN. Cellulose-retarded nitroglycerin and isosorbide dinitrate arrested or improved existing anginal symptoms (in 3 cases with oral Synchron nitroglycerin, in 1 with ISDN).

Discussion

The therapeutic efficacy of nitroglycerin in the management of angina pectoris symptoms [3, 8, 11, 13] and acute myocardial failure [2, 4, 5, 10] is undisputed. A further indication might be the combined use with beta-adrenoceptor blockers in the case of refractory angina and concomitant heart failure, as the specific properties of nitroglycerin counteract the negative inotropic effects of the beta blockers [5, 7]. The clinical effectiveness of nitroglycerin is due to a reduction in myocardial O_2 demand and relief of heart performance [1, 2, 12]. Cellulose-retarded nitroglycerin can result in a sustained release of the active agent during the gastrointestinal passage with a corresponding increase in the duration of action. According to *Volkmer and Hochrein* [10], even as little as 6.5 mg nitroglycerin in the formulation lowered the pulmonary artery pressure for 4–6 h. With this dose *Amsterdam* et al. [1] noted a reduction in left ventricular end-diastolic pressure up to 4 h, while on the basis of general clinical data *Strumza* et al. [9], and *Hirshleifer* [6] even assumed an effect of 8 h and longer.

In this study 10–20 mg of an oral Synchron nitroglycerin preparation also brought about a sustained drop in pulmonary pressure values and in right atrial influx pressure which could be defined as a definite drug effect for altogether 6 h. Even after 8 h the values were very much lower than the baseline values. However, when measured against the standard of the placebo groups these differences could not definitely be interpreted as a nitroglycerin effect. The higher dosage form with 20 mg cellulose-retarded nitroglycerin caused a significant decrease in cardiac output which lasted for 3 h and was essentially due to a reduction in cardiac preload. Heart rate tended to increase, while systemic arterial pressure showed no changes of a specific tendency. The changes in the left ventricular stroke work index and pulmonary artery wedge pressure led to a nitroglycerin-induced displacement of the work point on the heart function curve to a more favorable hemodynamic area and lasted up to 6 or 7 h. Maximum action was recorded between the 1st and 4th hour post application and the plasma concentration of nitroglycerin reached its peak in the 2nd hour. The correlation between concentration and hemodynamic response, however, could not be established as the test group was very small at this stage. Under exercise stress conditions, definite nitroglycerin effects could only be detected in the 4th hour, and not in the 8th. In respect of hemodynamic effects 10–20 mg of oral Synchron nitroglycerin were equipotent to a dose of 40 mg isosorbide dinitrate.

Cellulose-retarded nitroglycerin proved to be a highly effective substance with a definite, long-acting hemodynamic response of 6 h at rest and during exercise.

References

1 Amsterdam, E.A.; Awan, N.; Tonkon, M.; Wampold, D.; DeMaria, A.N.; Hason, D.T.: Sustained reduction of elevated left ventricular filling pressure in cardiac failure by oral sustained nitroglycerin. Circulation *51/52:* suppl. II, 150 (1975).

2 Bussmann, W.-D.: Nitroglycerin bei Herzinfarkt. Von der Kontraindikation zur Indikation. Dt. med. Wschr. *105:* 1551 (1980).

3 Cole, S.L.; Kaye, H.: Antianginal effects of oral controlled release nitroglycerin (GTN) in patients with coronary artery disease (CAD). Double blind randomized, multiple crossover study. Clin. Res. *23:* 177 (1975).

4 Hochrein, H.; Lehmann, H.-U.; Witt, E.; Traue, P.: Invasive methods for assessing the bioavailability of nitroglycerin in compensated and decompensated coronary heart disease. Br. J. clin. Pract., suppl. 12, p. 46 (1981).

5 Hillen, H.; Witt, E.; Lehmann, H.-U.; Hochrein, H.: Nitroglycerin, Dopamin und deren kombinierte Anwendung bei schwerer Myokardinsuffizienz. Intensivmed. *18:* 11 (1981).

6 Hirshleifer, I.: Peripheral hemodynamic effect of oral controlled release nitroglycerin in man. Curr. ther. Res. *15:* 158 (1973).

7 Lehmann, H.-U.; Oeff, M.; Witt, E.; Hochrein, H.: Die Behandlung des akuten Myokardinfarktes mit Betarezeptorenblockern. II. Hämodynamische Effekte von Propranolol mit und ohne Kombinationstherapie mit Nitroglycerin. Z. Kardiol. *70:* 748 (1981).

8 Needleman, P.; Lang, S.; Johnson, E.M.: Organic nitrites: relationship between biotransformation and rational angina pectoris therapy. J. Pharmac. exp. Ther. *181:* 489 (1972).

9 Strumza, P.; Rigaud, M.; Mechmeche, R.; Rocha, P.; Baudet, M.; Bardet, J.; Bourdarias, J.P.: Prolonged hemodynamic effects (12 hours) of orally administered sustained-release nitroglycerin. Am. J. Cardiol. *43:* 272 (1979).

10 Volkmer, F.; Hochrein, H.: Wirkung von Retard-Nitroglycerin auf den Pulmonalarteriendruck bei koronarer Herzkrankheit. Dt. med. Wschr. *102:* 1458 (1977).

11 Wendkos, M.H.; Meshulam, N.: Comparative effects of placebo and sustained-release nitroglycerin in anginal subjects. J. clin. Pharm. *13:* 160 (1973).

12 Winsor, I.; Berger, H.J.: Oral nitroglycerin as a prophylactic antianginal drug. Am. Heart J. *90:* 611 (1975).

13 Yap, S.K.; Rhodes, C.T.; Fung, H.L.: Quality control and drug analysis. Am. J. Hosp. Pharm. *32:* 1039 (1975).

H.-U. Lehmann, MD, III. Medizinische Klinik, Rudolf-Virchow-Krankenhaus, Augustenburger Platz 1, D-1000 Berlin 65

Discussion

Chairmen: *U. Gleichmann* and *N. Reichek*

Bussmann: You demonstrated 3 cases with the very low plasma levels. Did they have sufficient hemodynamic effects?

Lehmann: The astonishing phenomenon is that one person with a very marked hemodynamic reaction had a serum concentration of 0.3 mg/ml. Basically it were not those patients with a very high nitroglycerin level in the blood serum who had a strong action in hemodynamics.

Bussmann: May I ask Dr. *Fung:* Do you think that in some patients such low levels and in others nicely high levels are possible?

Fung: The variability would be expected and actually would be anticipated based on the fact that this is a very highly cleared drug. And this is almost characteristic of any drug that is subjected to extensive first-pass metabolism, because different individuals may have different capacity to metabolize the drug. I also have maybe a partial response to the false-positive question. It obviously is very disturbing to have false positives. One doesn't know where it comes from. I think the only way to do it is to make sure that you ran blanks, to make sure that samples before dosing are taken so that, whatever concentration there is, it is corrected. And to make sure that the assay laboratory and the personnel who handle the samples take extreme care to avoid any cross-labelling of samples that may eventually result in false positives. This assay in terms of specificity is as specific as any other assay. No chemical method is always 100% foolproof because you rely on the chromatogram and something could co-chromatograph with it. The only thing that you could use is a gas-chromatograph combined with a mass spectrometer, so that with every sample that you do, you confirm the molecular weight of the sample. There is essentially no other way to do this. But I think it is a great idea for you to throw in random samples of blanks or of low concentration just to check the validity. I think this is a fantastic practice for validating the assay.

Bussmann: You said that with oral nitroglycerin there is a big first-pass effect. We have always seen a strong first-pass effect after oral isosorbide dinitrate, but when we looked at blood levels with high doses, we found reasonable blood levels. Is the first-pass effect for these two drugs different or is it in the end the same thing? Do we only have to increase the dose?

Fung: I think, if we say extensive first-pass metabolism, it is a matter of degrees. Obviously many drugs are absorbed close to 100%, like theophylline, but many drugs are absorbed up to only 20 or 30%. And we then say that this latter class is subjected to extensive first-pass. I have not conducted a cross-over study in man, in which I give intravenous nitroglycerin and oral nitroglycerin to determine the exact first-pass metabolism. I have done that in animals and it showed that the first-pass metabolism is dose-dependent. And in man the oral bioavailability of nitroglycerin may also be dose-dependent. With ISDN we do have human data which we obtained when we crossed-over oral administration and intravenous administration. Our experience is that the oral administration of isosorbide dinitrate is quite bioavailable: it could go anywhere from individual to individual say from 10 to 70% compared with intravenous administration. So it is not completely first-pass.

Adv. Pharmacother., vol. 1, pp. 194–203 (Karger, Basel 1982)

Efficacy and Dosage of Oral Synchron Nitroglycerin in Patients with Coronary Heart Disease

A. Konrads[a], *W. Hummerich*[a], *H. Strödter*[b], *R.-R. Dries*[c]

[a] Medizinische Universitäts-Poliklinik, Köln; [b] Innere Medizin III (Kardiologie), Universität Köln, Köln; [c] Dr. Thiemann GmbH, Klinische Forschung, Lünen, FRG

Introduction

In the last 100 years [1] nitroglycerin has become a well-established drug in acute angina pectoris treatment. Furthermore, recent studies have shown that oral application of controlled release nitroglycerin contributes favorably to the long-term treatment of coronary heart diseases [2, 3]. However, a sufficiently high dosage has to be selected because of the extensive hepatic metabolism [4]. This study is designed to examine the efficacy of oral nitroglycerin as a controlled release, Synchron formulation administered in three different dosage forms to patients with coronary heart disease.

Patients and Methods

36 patients (28 male, 8 female; mean age 52 years) were included in the study which was designed as a single-blind prospective trial (fig. 1). After a selection phase of 1 week with the patients being examined as to their satisfying certain criteria for admission to the study and the determination of baseline values for the various parameters prior to treatment, a titration phase of a maximum of 3 weeks followed to select the individual optimum dosage by serial administration. We started with an initial dose of 2 × 2.6 mg daily and, depending on symptoms during the weekly follow-up, the dosage was maintained or increased to 2 × 6.5 mg or even 2 × 10 mg daily. Thus, the patients were allocated to three dosage groups: group I (5.2 mg/d) 8 patients, group II (13 mg/day) 15 patients and group III (20 mg/day) 13 patients. The drug phase extended over a period of 7 weeks in which the patients received the individual dosage selected during the titration phase. Follow-up examinations (clinical examination, exercise testing according to *Kaltenbach* [5], standard biochemical parameters) were done at the end of the selection phase as well as after 3 and/or 7 weeks of test drug administration (fig. 1). The Freiburg List of Complaints – Repetition Form was used to determine subjective symptoms prior to and during the drug

phase. The protocol included blood taking for determination of renin and vasopressin plasma concentrations during the selection phase and 3 and 7 weeks after drug administration, these results are published in detail elsewhere [6].

Patients had to satisfy the following criteria to be admitted to the study: characteristic exercise-induced, retrosternal pain; positive exercise ECG with ST-segment depression of at least 0.1 mV; positive response to acute application of nitroglycerin. Treatment with other antianginal drugs (such as beta-blockers, calcium antagonists, long-acting nitrates) was discontinued 2 weeks prior to the study. 10 out of 36 patients had undergone coronary arteriography; this, however, was not a precondition for admission to the study. Excluded were patients with severe cardiovascular disorders 6 months prior to the study (myocardial infarction, congestive heart failure, arrhythmias, etc.) or with other severe physiological disorders. No patient received a concomitant therapy with analgetics or psychopharmacological drugs.

The frequency of daily anginal attacks and the number of sublingual nitroglycerin caps necessary for relief of attacks were recorded separately.

Results

Mean duration of the titration phase was 14 days. During this period an overall significant reduction in anginal frequency and acute nitroglycerin administration was noted. Comparing the three dosage groups at baseline showed a significant correlation between dose size and severity of coronary heart disease: Effort tolerance ($p < 0.01$), anginal frequency ($p < 0.001$), and number of nitroglycerin capsules ($p < 0.05$) differed significantly. The score sums of the Freiburg List of Complaints did not reveal any significant correlation with dose size.

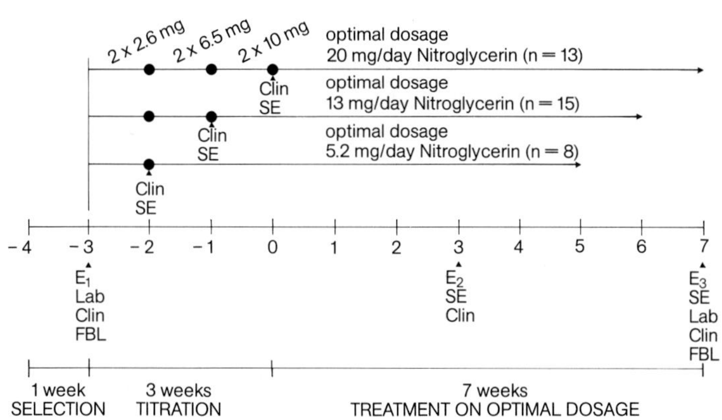

Fig. 1. Study design. FBL = Freiburg list of complaints; Clin = clinical checkup; Lab = laboratory data; SE = side effect rating; E = ergometry.

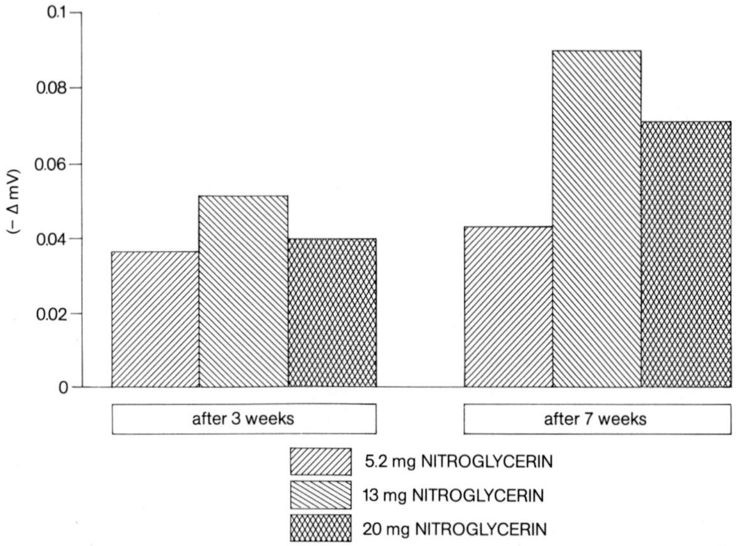

Fig. 2. Improvement (decrease) of ST-segment depression after 3 or 7 weeks of nitroglycerin administration in three different dosage groups. Difference to baseline.

Exercise Testing. In comparing exercise tests after 3 or 7 weeks of drug administration to baseline values no statistically significant changes in heart rate and blood pressure could be noted. ST-segment depression diminished during the drug phase from 0.168 to 0.124 mV after 3 weeks ($p = 0.020$) and from 0.179 to 0.107 mV after 7 weeks ($p < 0.001$). Figure 2 shows the diminution of ST-segment depression in the three dosage groups. Overall exercise tolerance is increased. This is reflected in the increase in mean intraindividual workload ($p = 0.052$) after 7 weeks and in an increase in the duration of exercise ($p = 0.064$ after 3 weeks and $p = 0.170$ after 7 weeks). Consequently, effort tolerance (fig. 3) increases as well ($p = 0.085$ after 3 weeks and $p = 0.053$ after 7 weeks). After 4 and 7 weeks of drug administration in 3 and 4 patients exercise-induced anginal symptoms are no longer observed in contrast to the selection phase. The time of anginal onset has only slightly changed during 3 weeks. After 7 weeks, however, we find a significant increase from 284 to 397 s ($p = 0.024$) for intraindividually comparable cases. In group I with the lowest dosage, additional cardiac arrhythmias were observed in 1 patient and in group II in 2 patients. In group III (20 mg/day) arrhythmias did not subside in 1 patient, and were no longer recorded in 2 patients during the study; in 1 patient of group II normalization of this disorder was observed.

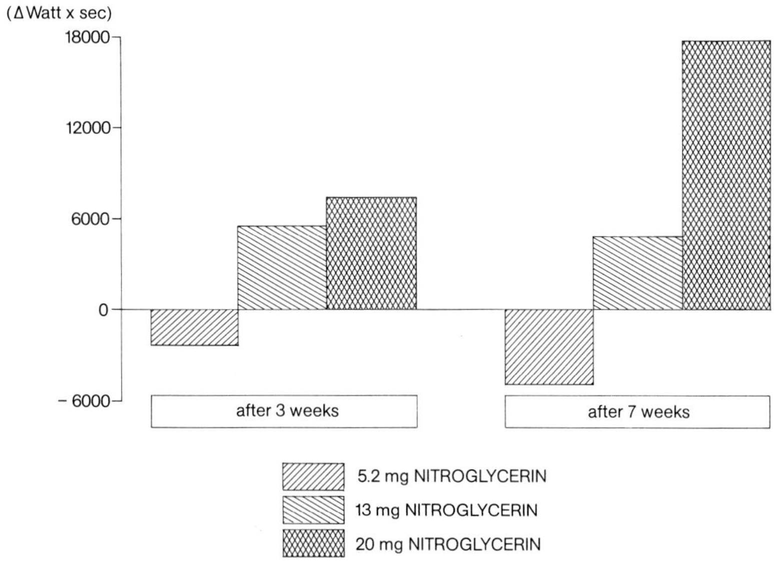

Fig. 3. Increase in effort tolerance after 3 or 7 weeks of nitroglycerin administration in three different dosage groups. Difference to baseline.

Frequency of Angina pectoris and Dosage of Sublingual Nitroglycerin Caps. After 3 and 7 weeks anginal frequency was significantly reduced against baseline during the selection phase ($p < 0.001$) with a more pronounced improvement after 7 weeks of medication than after 3 weeks ($p < 0.034$). All three dosage groups had a reduction in the mean weekly frequency of anginal episodes (fig. 4, 5). Figure 5 shows a dose-related improvement reflecting the direct correlation between the severity of the disorder and the individual dose size. There is also a significant reduction in the sublingual nitroglycerin dosage for relief of anginal attacks after 3 and 7 weeks of medication ($p < 0.001$ respectively). Here again the strongest effect was noted in the highest dosage group in relation to the severity of the disease (fig. 6).

Side Effects. Patients noted as side effects headache and a sense of fullness of the head; in 1 case, medication had to be discontinued due to severe headache. In another patient a relation between nitroglycerin application and untoward effects such as heartburn and nausea was assumed. No further relevant side effects were noted. Among 22 patients examined in Cologne for

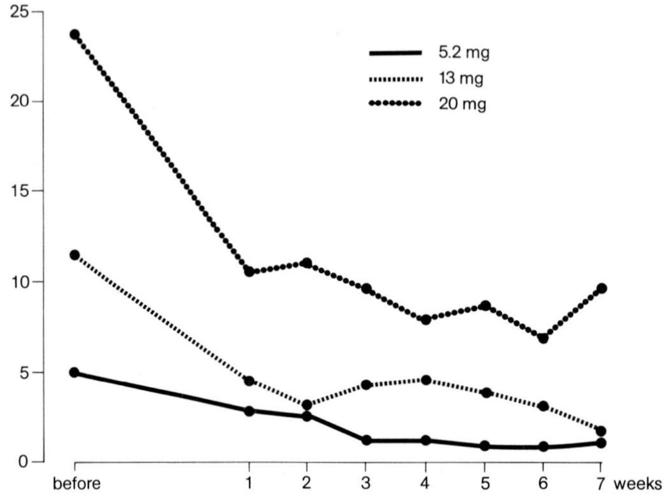

Fig. 4. Mean frequency of angina pectoris attacks per week before and after 7 weeks of nitroglycerin medication in three dosage groups.

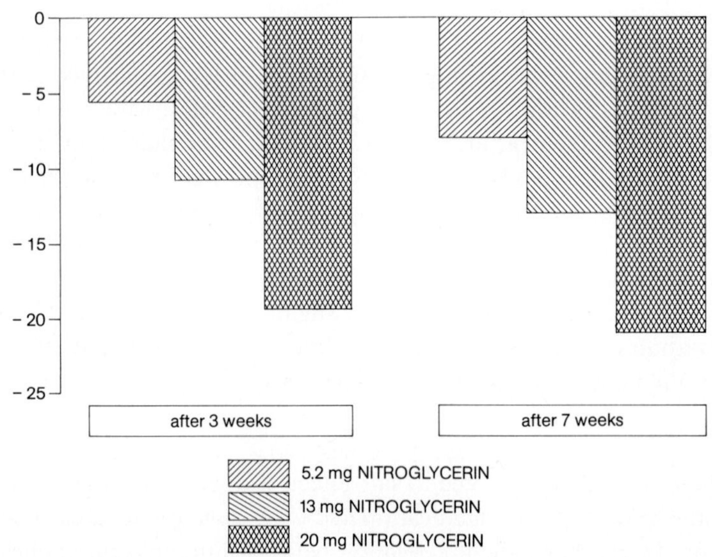

Fig. 5. Reduction in mean anginal frequency per week after 3 or 7 weeks of nitroglycerin medication in three dosage groups. Difference to baseline.

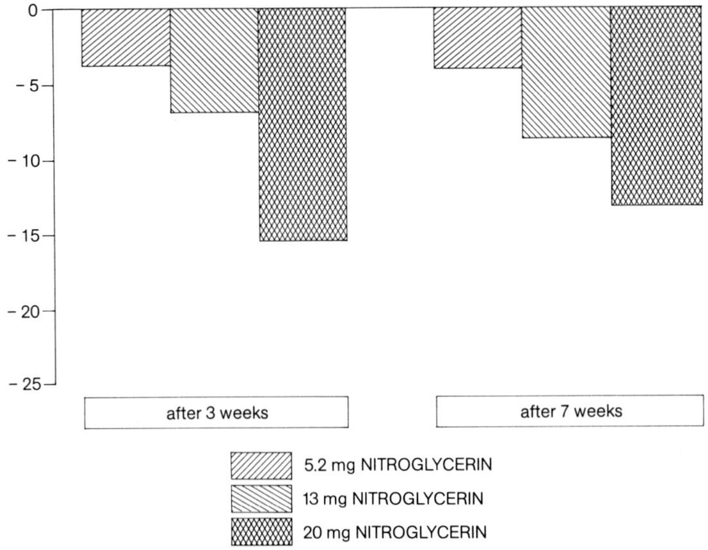

Fig. 6. Reduction in the mean sublingual nitroglycerin dosage per week to relieve an acute anginal attack after 3 or 7 weeks of nitroglycerin administration in three dosage groups. Difference to baseline.

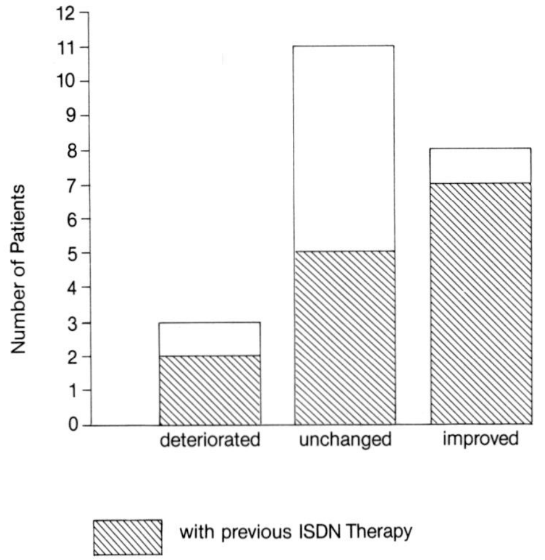

Fig. 7. Changes in the severity of headaches after 7 weeks of nitroglycerin treatment in comparison to baseline.

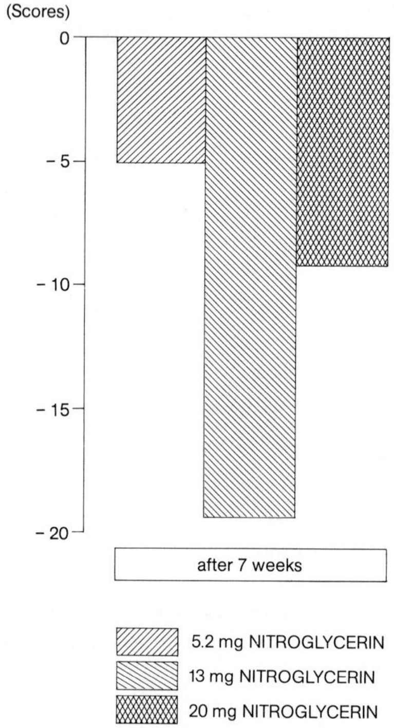

Fig. 8. Reduction (improvement) in the score sum of the Freiburg List of Complaints after 7 weeks of nitroglycerin administration in three dosage groups compared to baseline.

this study, the severity of headaches was – after evaluation of the Freiburg List of Complaints – aggravated in 3 patients, unchanged in 11 and improved in 8 after 7 weeks of medication against baseline of the selection phase. 7 of the 8 patients with an improvement had previously had isosorbide dinitrate (fig. 7). Overall, the Freiburg List of Complaints – parameters revealed a statistically significant improvement in the individual state of health of the total study population, with regard to the subscores: general health ($p = 0.01$), cardiovascular system ($p < 0.001$), gastrointestinal tract ($p = 0.026$) and the sum of symptoms ($p = 0.005$) with a positive maximum effect in group II with the intermediate dosage (fig. 8). There were no statistically significant differences among the dosage groups I through III. During nitroglycerin administration clinical and biochemical parameters did not show any relevant changes.

Discussion

During the 7 weeks of medication with oral Synchron nitroglycerin, patients with coronary heart disease showed a significant improvement in subjective and objective parameters in comparison to the selection phase without any antianginal therapy. As a subjective parameter we used the frequency of anginal episodes and, directly related to that, the number of sublingual nitroglycerin capsules required for anginal relief as another variable. Referring to the patients' records we could show that anginal frequency and thus also sublingual nitroglycerin dosage diminished significantly during application of oral Synchron nitroglycerin. Drug action showed a significant relation to dose size. As objective parameters changes in exercise testing were used. We detected a reduction of ST-segment depression and an increase in workload and exercise tolerance. These findings are confirmed by other authors who record hemodynamic effects 6–8 h after a single oral application of this nitroglycerin formulation, thus corroborating the efficacy of oral Synchron nitroglycerin [7–9].

In the present study we tried to establish the individual optimum dose in a titration phase. We started with a low initial dosage of 2×2.6 mg daily and increased up to a maximum of 2×10 mg/d on the basis of subjective information of the patient on the frequency of anginal attacks at the weekly follow-up examination. In this procedure with its orientation to the patients' symptoms, 80% required the higher dosage, i.e. 13 or 20 mg/day. This type of dose selection was indicated by the fact that, during our long-term treatment, no patient required another dose adaptation because of increase in anginal frequency. Comparison of dosage groups at baseline showed that the required dose size was related to the intensity of symptoms as a direct correlation between dosage and anginal frequency was detected in the selection phase. Consequently, the reduction in anginal frequency and nitroglycerin requirements were dose-related as well. Whether a further dose size increase to more than 20 mg/day would result in additional action was not tested. It also remains to be clarified to what extent the tolerance factor affects long-term therapy with nitroglycerin [10]. *Davidov and Mroczek* [11] demonstrated similar results from a double-blind study over 6 months on a long-acting nitrate of similar or higher dosage (19.5–39 mg/d). In acute studies lower doses of long-acting oral nitroglycerin drugs (2.6–7.8 mg) have shown their efficacy in hemodynamic [12–16] and exercise test studies [17].

As predicted, the results of the physical examination and relevant biochemical parameters did not show any drug-related pathological changes during therapy. Side effects were recorded by asking the patients during therapy and by checking the patients statements against the Freiburg List of Complaints. For a long time it has been known that headaches are the most frequent subjectively felt side effect under acute or long-term treatment with nitrates. In our study nitroglycerin medication had to be discontinued in 1 case only because of severe headaches. In some other cases the intensity of headaches was graded as less severe than at baseline. The evaluation of the Freiburg List of Complaints showed a significant improvement of general health and of gastrointestinal or cardiovascular symptoms. Reduction in incidence and intensity of cardiovascular symptoms can be attributed to the test agent directly whereas a reduction in other symptoms should rather be attributed to indirect effects.

We conclude that oral Synchron nitroglycerin is a highly effective, well tolerated, controlled release nitrate, administered twice a day in doses of 13–20 mg/day, with few side effects and is well suited for long-term treatment of patients with coronary heart disease.

Acknowledgement

We would like to thank Prof. Dr. *G. Fricke* and Priv. Doz. (Asst. Prof.) Dr. *H. Mattern*, of the Universitäts-Poliklinik Bonn for their participation in the clinical studies. We are also indebted to Dr. *J. Schnitker*, Institut für angewandte Statistik, Bielefeld, for the statistical evaluation of the corresponding data.

References

1 Murrell, W.: Nitroglycerin as a remedy for angina pectoris. Lancet *i:* 80–81 (1879).

2 Abrams, J.: Usefullness of long-acting nitrates in cardiovascular disease. Am. J. Med. *64:* 183–186 (1978).

3 Kaverina, N.V.; Chumburidze, V.B.: Antianginal drugs. Pharmacol. Ther. *4:* 109–153 (1979).

4 Needleman, P.; Harkey, A.B.: Role of endogenous glutathione in the metabolism of glyceryl trinitrate by isolated perfused rat liver. Biochem. Pharmacol. *20:* 1867–1876 (1971).

5 Kaltenbach, M.: Medikamentöse Therapie der koronaren Herzkrankheit. Arzneimittel-Forsch. *27:* 703–707 (1977).

6 Hummerich, W.; Konrads, A.; Wambach, G.; Meurer, K.A.; Dries, R.-R.; Langbehn, A.-F.: This volume.

7 Hochrein, H.; Lehmann, H.U.; Witt, E.; Traue, P.: Invasive methods for assessing the bioavailability of nitroglycerin in compensated and decompensated coronary heart disease. Br. J. clin. Pract. *12:* suppl., pp. 46–49 (1981).

8 Erb, R.J.: This volume.

9 Lehmann, H.-U.; Witt, E.; Traue, P.; Hochrein, H.: This volume.
10 Abrams, J.: Nitrate tolerance and dependence. Am. Heart J. *99:* 113–123 (1980).
11 Davidov, M.E.; Mroczek, W.J.: The effects of sustained release nitroglycerin capsules on angina frequency and exercise capacity. Angiology *28:* 181–189 (1977).
12 Hirshleifer, I.: Peripheral hemodynamic effects of oral controlled-release nitroglycerin (nitrong) in man. Curr. ther. Res. *15:* 158–164 (1973).
13 Hirshleifer, I.: Nitroglycerin: clinical pharmacological effects of form and route of administration. Curr. ther. Res. *15:* 616–623 (1973).
14 Winsor, T.; Berger, H.: Oral nitroglycerin as a prophylactic antianginal drug. Clinical, physiologic, and statistical evidence of efficacy based on a three-phase experimental design. Am. Heart J. *90:* 611 (1975).
15 Volkmer, F.; Hochrein, H.: Wirkung von Retard-Nitroglycerin auf den Pulmonalarteriendruck bei koronarer Herzkrankheit. Dt. med. Wschr. *102:* 1458–1460 (1977).
16 Strumza, P.; Rigaud, M.; Mechmeche, R.; Rocha, P.; Baudet, M.; Bardet, J.; Bourdarias, J.-P.: Prolonged hemodynamic effects (12 hours) or orally administered sustained-release nitroglycerin. Am. J. Cardiol. *43:* 272–277 (1979).
17 Wendkos, M.H.; Meshulam, N.: Comparative effects of placebo and sustained-release nitroglycerin in anginal subjects. J. clin. Pharm. *13:* 160–166 (1973).

A. Konrads, MD, Medizinische Universitäts-Poliklinik, Joseph-Stelzmann-Strasse 9, D-5000 Köln 41 (FRG)

Discussion

Chairmen: *U. Gleichmann* and *N. Reichek*

Wagner: What were the criteria for increasing the dosage during the titration phase or for not increasing the dosage?

Konrads: Well as I said, criteria for increasing the dosage were the clinical parameters. This selection of the dose was just related to the symptoms of the patient and the clinical checkup during the weekly intervals when we controlled patients during the titration period.

Reichek: Perhaps I might make a comment. I have no controlled data. However, with the buccal preparation our outpatient trial has inherited many problem patients. I think 6 of the 17 patients we have tried chronically on the buccal preparation had failed or been intolerant of isosorbide treatment because of intolerable headache. Only 1 of these had to be dropped from buccal treatment because of headache. We've had the impression that there may be a real difference. I think it will be terribly difficult to design any adequate evaluation to sort that out, but our impression is that there may be a real difference, at least, for the buccal preparation.

Bussmann: There is a good protocol to investigate side effects like headache: in volunteers who get headache in 50%. During our last meeting here ISDN was compared with 5-mononitrate. The headache incidence was exactly the same. Oral nitroglycerin reduces anginal attacks in a dose-dependent fashion. Dr. *Schneider* from our group demonstrated a dose-dependent improvement of ST-segment depression and at the same time a dose-dependent decrease in frequency of anginal attacks for both ISDN and GTN.

Adv. Pharmacother., vol. 1, pp. 204–209 (Karger, Basel 1982)

Dose-Response Relationship of Oral Nitroglycerin in the Treatment of Coronary Heart Disease

W. Schneider, B. Stahl, M. Kaltenbach, W.-D. Bussmann

Zentrum der Inneren Medizin, Abteilung für Kardiologie, Klinikum der Johann Wolfgang Goethe-Universität, Frankfurt a.M., BRD

Introduction

For more than 100 years nitrates have been used for the treatment of angina pectoris [6]. The potent but rapidly subsiding antianginal effect of nitroglycerin led to the development of organic nitrates with a longer duration of action [4]. The presently available, long-acting nitrates are isosorbide dinitrate, pentaerythritol tetranitrate, erythrityl tetranitrate, trolnitrate, etc.; most of them administered as oral delivery systems. In the last few years the high efficacy of sublingual nitroglycerin has initiated tests to develop a long-acting delivery form for this drug by changing the formulation. In oral administration the major problem stems from the strong hepatic first pass metabolism this agent is subject to. In the first clinical trials, preparations with a 3- to 8-fold higher nitroglycerin quantity than the conventional sublingual cap (0.8 mg) and a gastrointestinal sustained release of the drug gave hope of prolonged antianginal activity. Nitroglycerin is either bound to carrier molecules (e.g., polymerized cellulose) or incorporated into microcapsules. The introduction of oral slow-release nitroglycerin forms raised questions on the magnitude of action, i.e., antianginal potency and duration of action. This would finally answer the question whether nitroglycerin might provide a rational long-term treatment for angina pectoris. These problems will be studied in the work presented here. Besides the evaluation of the dose-response relationship in four different nitroglycerin dose sizes, the respective efficacy over a period of 6 h is assessed as well.

Methods

We have studied 12 male patients between 40 and 65 years of age with angiographically documented coronary heart disease (at least 70% occlusion in one or more major coronary arteries). In none of the patients was the coronary heart disease accompanied by other significant diseases. All patients complained of exercise-induced angina pectoris with an average anginal frequency of five attacks per week. In all patients the exercise ECG showed a reproducible ischemic reaction with an ST segment depression of more than 1 mm. Prior to the study all other cardioactive drugs were discontinued. Informed consent was acquired from all patients. The study was designed as a double-blind, 5-fold cross-over intraindividual protocol.

After a 2-day premedication phase, placebo and nitroglycerin bound to modified hydroxypropylmethylcellulose (Synchron-GTN) were orally administered at the same time on 5 different days, with a control interval of 2–4 days at a dosage of 2.6, 6.5, 10, and 20 mg nitroglycerin. The test samples were physically indistinguishable.

The 20-mg dose was administered as two 10-mg tablets and placebo was provided as tablets identical to the 2.6-, 6.5- and 10-mg active dose.

The noninvasive measurement of blood pressure and heart rate in an upright (standing) and supine position preceded drug administration. A 12-lead standard ECG was recorded at rest. On each study day, exercise performance was evaluated 1 h prior to the administration of the test agent (control test), as well as 30 min, 3 h, and 6 h after it. Exercise testing was carried out with the two-step test at constant individual submaximal workload. The normal exercise time was 6 min, the rest period always 5 min. For a quantitative evaluation of the ischemic reaction, ST segment depression was measured in millimeters using the lead with maximum ECG changes; mean value was computed out of five beats for each minute. During and after exercise, the ST depression was added minute by minute and the total ST segment depression was expressed numerically and percentagewise in comparison to the control value.

Besides the time of beginning of anginal pain during stress testing was documented during all trials.

Data were compared using Student's t test.

Results

Demonstration of a Dose-Dependent Antianginal Effect of Orally Administered Nitroglycerin

In our control test, the mean sum of ST segment depression was 10.7 mm during the exercise and rest period. 30 min after administration of placebo no significant changes occurred as compared to control (10.2 vs. 10.7 mm; table I, fig. 1). 30 min after administration of 2.6 mg nitroglycerin, the sum of ST segment depression was significantly reduced to 8.01 mm, corresponding to a 25% reduction in comparison to control data. After 6.5 mg nitroglycerin, the ST segment depression reduction was 6.4 mm, corresponding to a 40% reduction as compared to control. The respective value after 10 mg nitro-

Table I. Sum of ST segment depressions during and after load in patients with coronary heart disease (n = 6) under different doses of nitroglycerin (GTN, mm)

Medication	A	B	C	D
Placebo	10.88 ± 4.05	10.40 ± 4.63	10.71 ± 4.84	11.98 ± 5.50
2.6 mg GTN	10.68 ± 4.21	8.01 ± 4.29	7.97 ± 4.68	9.92 ± 4.24
6.5 mg GTN	10.48 ± 4.28	6.38 ± 3.45	6.56 ± 3.96	8.54 ± 4.35
10 mg GTN	11.12 ± 4.48	4.66 ± 2.90	4.58 ± 3.30	7.30 ± 4.97
20 mg GTN	10.53 ± 4.14	2.66 ± 1.98	2.59 ± 2.03	5.31 ± 3.61

A: Ergometry prior to drug intake (pretest); B: ergometry 30 min after drug intake; C: ergometry 3 h after drug intake; D: ergometry 6 h after drug intake (mean values ± standard deviation).

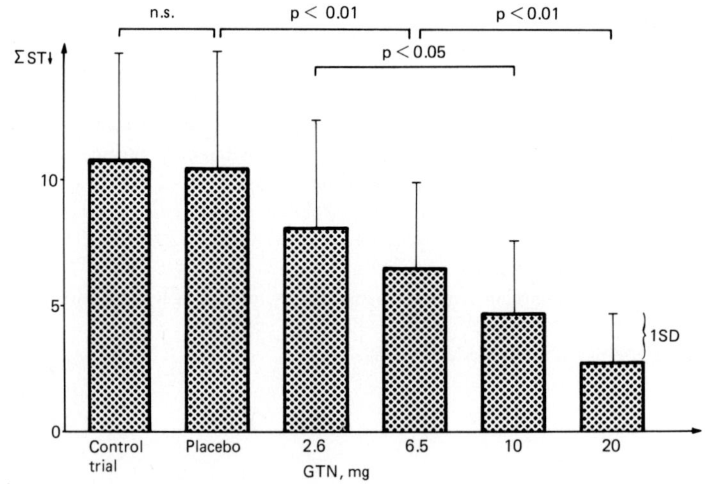

Fig. 1. Sum of ST segment depressions during load and recovery phase in patients with coronary heart disease (n = 12) after different oral doses of nitroglycerin (GTN). Mean values ± SD.

glycerin was 4.7 mm (equivalent to a reduction by 56%). The oral administration of 20 mg of the active agent produced a reduction in the sum of ST segment depression by 75% (2.7 mm) after 30 min.

Duration of Antianginal Action after Oral Nitroglycerin

After administration of 6.5, 10 and 20 mg, the mean values of the sum of ST segment depression at 3 and after 20 mg even at 6 h differed statistically

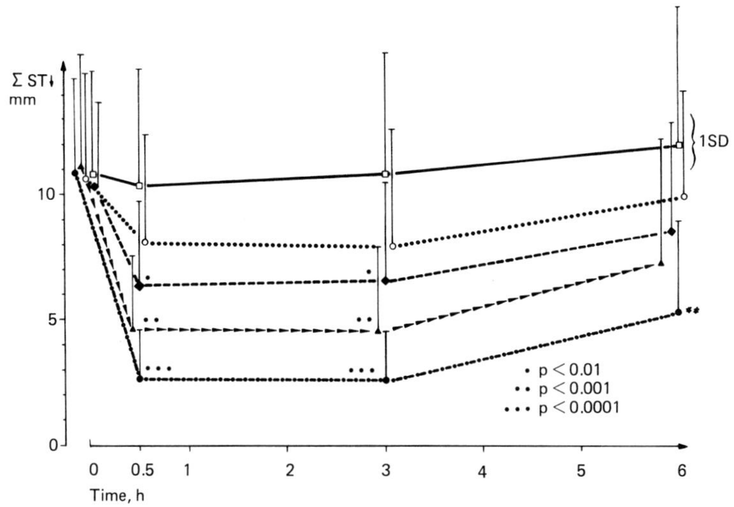

Fig. 2. Sum of ST segment depressions during and after ergometric load, 30 min after oral application of placebo and nitroglycerin (GTN). □ = Placebo; ○ = 2.6 mg GTN; ■ = 6.5 mg GTN; ▲ = 10.0 mg GTN; ● = 20.0 mg GTN. 0 h = Ergometry prior to application of drug or placebo. Mean values ± SD, n = 12.

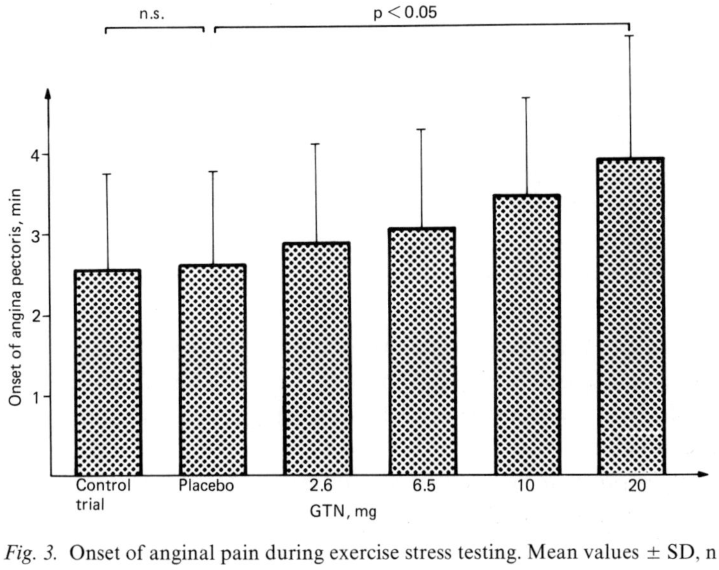

Fig. 3. Onset of anginal pain during exercise stress testing. Mean values ± SD, n = 12.

significant from control values (table I, fig. 2). The onset of anginal pain during stress testing did not differ between the control (2.5 min) and placebo trial (2.6 min) (mean values). The onset of symptoms was delayed by the various doses of nitroglycerin: 2.6 mg GTN, 2.9 min; 6.5 mg GTN, 3.1 min; 10 mg GTN, 3.5 min; 20 mg GTN, 3.9 min (fig. 3).

Side Effects

The administration of the active drug and placebo was tolerated well by all patients without any significant adverse effects.

Discussion

The potent antianginal efficacy of sublingual nitroglycerin has led to the development of other delivery forms for this drug with a sustained prophylactic effect. In our study an oral delivery system was used. The active agent nitroglycerin is incorporated in a pharmacologically inert polymer substance (modified hydroxypropylmethylcellulose) providing constant drug release. Intestinal absorption of nitroglycerin is assured [5]. The determination of plasma levels showed that after oral administration of 7.5 mg nitroglycerin (in microcapsules) a peak occurred after 3 h (4.82 ng/ml). The plasma level falls below 1.0 ng/ml as late as 8 h thereafter [2]. Hemodynamic studies showed that the 5- and 7.5-mg doses of oral nitroglycerin produced a reduction in central venous pressure and in left and right ventricular filling pressures beyond 8 h [3]. Our results give objective evidence of a prolonged antianginal effect after a sufficiently high nitroglycerin dose lasting for at least 6 h after a single dose of 20 mg. Digital plethysmographic studies confirmed a similar duration of action even in administering the lower dose of 2.6 mg nitroglycerin [10]. During chronic administration of 3 × 6.5 mg nitroglycerin *Davidov and Mroczek* [1] demonstrated a clear reduction in anginal frequency and, during exercise testing, a prolonged exercise duration from 5.7 to 8.5 min in their patients. Identical results were reported by *Winsor and Berger* [9] demonstrating a reduction in the frequency of anginal attacks during chronic administration over 6 months with 3 × 2.6 mg nitroglycerin as well as a delayed occurrence of chest pain during exercise to angina pectoris, compared to placebo.

A major problem in the use of nitrates for the treatment of coronary heart disease focusses on the correlation between higher efficacy and higher dosage. While a good dose-response relation was described for hemodynamic effects – reduction in blood pressure – by nitrates during acute but not chronic administration [8], we could demonstrate a dose-dependent improvement of the ST segment depression in our studies with isosorbide dinitrate as a not controlled release preparation for a dose range of 2.6–20 mg. If we use the ST segment depression improvement in the exercise ECG (in %) as a basis for comparing the efficacy of isosorbide dinitrate and nitroglycerin, the following oral dose sizes seem to be equipotent:

20 mg isosorbide dinitrate – 6.5 mg nitroglycerin (reduction in ischemic reaction by 40%); 40 mg isosorbide dinitrate – 10 mg nitroglycerin (reduction in ischemic reaction by 50%); 80 mg isosorbide dinitrate – 20 mg nitroglycerin (reduction in ischemic reaction by 70%).

The fact that a dose-response relationship could be demonstrated for a 'slow-release' drug is a strong argument for the efficacy of this drug.

References

1 Davidov, M.E.; Mrozcek, W.J.: Effect of sustained-release nitroglycerin capsules on anginal frequency and exercise capacity: a double blind evaluation. Angiology *28:* 181–189 (1977).

2 Girre, C.; Crouzette, J.; Fournier, P.E.; Koch, H.: Taux plasmatiques de nitroglycérine après administration orale et percutanée. Nouv. Presse méd. *34:* 2433–2436 (1980).

3 Gueret, P.; Rigaud, M.; Bardet, J.; Bourdarias, J.P.: Les effets hémodynamiques prolongés de l'administration orale de nitroglycérine encapsulée. Nouv. Presse méd. *34:* 2451–2454 (1980).

4 Krantz, J.C., Jr.; Corr, C.J.; Forman, S.E.; Cone, N.: Medianism and action of organic nitrates. J. Pharmac. exp. Ther. *70:* 323–327 (1940).

5 Krantz, J.C., Jr.; Lake, C.D.: The gastrointestinal absorption of organic nitrates. Am. J. Cardiol. *36:* 407–408 (1975).

6 Murrell, W.: Nitroglycerine as a remedy for angina pectoris. Lancet *i:* 80 (1879).

7 Schneider, W.; Stahl, B.; Kaltenbach, M.; Bussmann, W.-D.: Dosis-Wirkungsbeziehungen bei der Behandlung der koronaren Herzkrankheit mit Isosorbiddinitrat. Z. Kardiol. *70:* 321 (1981).

8 Thadani, U.; Manyari, D.; Parker, J.O.; Fung, H.-L.: Tolerance to the circulatory effects of oral isosorbide dinitrate of development and cross tolerance to glyceryl trinitrate. Circulation *61:* 526–535 (1980).

9 Winsor, W.; Berger, H.J.: Oral nitroglycerin as a prophylactic antianginal drug: clinical, physiologic, and statistic evidence of efficacy based on a three-phase experimental design. Am Heart J. *90:* 6111–626 (1975).

10 Winsor, T.; Kaye, H.; Mills, B.: Hemodynamic response of oral long-acting nitrates. Evidence of gastrointestinal absorption. Chest *62:* 407–413 (1972).

W. Schneider, MD, Zentrum der Inneren Medizin, Abteilung für Kardiologie, Klinikum der Johann Wolfgang Goethe-Universität, D-6000 Frankfurt a.M. (FRG)

Adv. Pharmacother., vol. 1, pp. 210–213 (Karger, Basel 1982)

Summary

W.-D. Bussmann

Center of Internal Medicine, Department of Cardiology, University Clinic of the Johann Wolfgang Goethe University, Frankfurt am Main, FRG

The presentations and discussions during the workshop enable us to make a summary of the two types of preparations: the buccal and oral form of Synchron nitroglycerin. By critical evaluation of pharmacokinetic, hemodynamic and exercise-electrocardiographic results many of the questions posed can now be answered.

The excellent overview by Dr. *Abrams* pointed out the variety of different indications of nitrates today.

Dr. *Fung* discussed the importance of the site of drug administration and sampling in assessing nitroglycerin plasma levels. This is of relevance for the interpretation of pharmacokinetics. Only 1% nitroglycerin is left in the plasma. A much larger amount was found in the venous, arterial and the surrounding tissues. There is some information about the pharmacokinetics of buccal nitroglycerin. In regard of oral nitroglycerin, however, sufficient pharmacokinetic information is lacking. A number of problems exist beside the first pass-effect, for example the absorption may well vary from patient to patient.

Dr. *Hummerich* demonstrated that nitroglycerin during acute or long-term treatment does not adversely affect the renin-angiotensin-aldosteron system.

Buccal or oral nitroglycerin needs a carrier which releases the drug continuously. This is due to the short half-life of nitroglycerin (5 min), when calculated from plasma levels. Dr. *Davis* demonstrated the concept of the controlled release Synchron tablet. He observed the passage of the oral and the behavior of the buccal tablet by ^{99}Tc pictures. In his studies there is a continuous release of active substance over 3 h for the buccal and 6 h for the oral form. This was confirmed by Dr. *Erb's* study with digital plethysmography.

There are several groups which have acquired recent clinical experience with the buccal form of nitroglycerin *(Langbehn, Windorfer, Bussmann,*

Kaiser, Ohlmeier, Reichek, Lichstein, and *Prager).* Only a few have experience with the oral form of nitroglycerin *(Lehmann, Erb, Schneider,* and *Konrads).*

With the buccal tablet in the mouth, the characteristic hemodynamic effects become evident within 30 s (Dr. *Langbehn*). These are a reduction of left ventricular filling pressure, a slight decline in systolic arterial pressure, and dilatation of the large coronary arteries (Dr. *Bussmann*). Plasma concentration reaches 1–2 ng/ml within 10 min. Higher levels were observed (10 ng/ml), when the buccal tablet was dissolved within a short time. There is a good dose-response relationship from 1.0 to 2.5 to 5.0 mg of buccal nitroglycerin. In contrast to sublingual nitroglycerin plasma levels remain high for at least 60 min or more as long as the buccal tablet is physically present. The 'nitroglycerin infusion' by the buccal tablet can be stopped by removing the drug. If the tablet was in place for a certain time and is removed or dissolved, it takes 1–2 h or longer before the hemodynamic parameters return to the control values. This discrepancy between the rapidly decreasing plasma concentration and the long-lasting therapeutic effects has a direct bearing on Dr. *Fung's* thesis: nitroglycerin remains in the vessel walls, especially in the veins, and in the tissue around the site of administration.

Dr. *Reichek* and Dr. *Lichstein* found that a buccal tablet is effective for about 3–5 h as measured by exercise duration studies.

Dr. *Prager* evaluated patients with cold-induced angina pectoris under normal everyday conditions and could demonstrate the acute prophylactic effect of 1 mg buccal Synchron nitroglycerin. Effective treatment of the acute attacks with 2.5 mg buccal nitroglycerin was possible within 1.5 min, nearly as rapidly as with sublingual nitroglycerin.

Dr. *Konrads* investigated the oral form of nitroglycerin in a titration study. The effective single dose is 6.5 mg. The 2.6-mg oral tablet is only effective in a few patients. Single oral doses up to 10 mg were used. About 80% of the patients needed the larger doses (6.5 or 10 mg b.i.d.). Dr. *Lehmann* demonstrated that the duration of action of a single oral dose of 10 and 20 mg was 6 h, according to the studies of Drs. *Davis* and *Erb.* Dr. *Schneider* from our group demonstrated a clear dose-response relationship following oral nitroglycerin: antianginal activity increased to a 75% decrease of ST-segment depression when the dose was augmented from 2.6 to 20 mg. This is comparable to a former study using oral ISDN in a dose range from 5 to 80 mg.

The following dose schedule can be employed: the average effective buccal dose is 2.5 mg, 3 or 4 times a day. This is a daily dose of 7.5–10 mg of buccal nitroglycerin.

The average effective oral dose is 6.5–10 or 20 mg, 2–4 times a day. This is a daily dose of 13–40, up to 80 mg orally.

Regarding the effect of the buccal and oral form of Synchron nitroglycerin we can *conclude* the following:

(1) Buccal and oral nitroglycerin are effective in treating patients with angina pectoris.

(2) The effective buccal dose is 2.5 mg, 3–4 times a day. Much larger doses are needed using the oral form.

(3) Effective plasma nitroglycerin concentrations can be achieved with the buccal tablet. These levels are comparable to blood levels achieved by intravenous infusion of nitroglycerin. Blood levels following the oral dose, however, seem to vary markedly. In some cases even with a good hemodynamic response plasma levels remain very low (average 0.1 ng/ml). Sufficient information cannot be gained at the moment.

(4) The buccal form of nitroglycerin is of real clinical value. It has a rapid onset, long-acting profile. The dissolution of the tablet takes 2–3 h dependent on the movement of the tablet in the mouth and the activation of the tablet by salivation and water contact. The duration of the hemodynamic action of the buccal tablet is 4–5 h. A study to assess patient compliance with the buccal type of application under chronic treatment conditions has yet to be undertaken. Case reports are encouraging. The buccal tablet therefore seems to be a flexible formulation which enables us to treat the acute attack and is appropriate for the acute and chronic prophylaxis of angina pectoris.

(5) The information about the oral form of nitroglycerin is insufficient up to now. The few studies presented show that it is possible to use the oral tablet in reducing the frequency of anginal attacks. The dose is 6.5–10 mg, and up to 20 mg twice a day. ST-segment depression during exercise can be reduced by 75% compared to placebo. Antianginal activity remains present for 6 h, especially when the large dose (20 mg) is used. It should theoretically be possible also to use the oral Synchron tablet during the attack as a buccal and then quickly swallow it to avoid peak plasma levels but to get the long-term effect.

(6) Up to now there have been no studies which compare pellet formulations with the Synchron system. The only marginal effectiveness of pellets may be due to the low dose used.

(7) Side effects like headaches seem to occur less often with buccal or oral Synchron nitroglycerin than with isosorbide dinitrate. However, this has not been investigated in the double-blind fashion.

Conclusions

In general, I would say that this workshop and this book dealt with something new. We have put together the new information on a new preparation of nitroglycerin: the *buccal* controlled release form. It has a rapid onset like sublingual nitroglycerin but stays much longer than sublingual nitroglycerin or sublingual isosorbide dinitrate. The duration of action is 4–5 h. Furthermore, the patient is able to interrupt his own 'nitroglycerin infusion'. Plasma levels are reasonable in the range of 0.5–2.5 ng/ml. The dose range is 1.0–2.5 mg 3–4 times a day. With 5.0 mg side effects like hypotension and tachycardia were seen in a few patients.

There are some problems with the buccal form of nitroglycerin which have not been solved yet. The compliance of patients to the tablet in the buccal region has not really been investigated. Encouraging case reports suggest that some of the patients prefer the buccal application to other oral dinitrates. A 3 times daily strategy seems to be sufficient in most cases.

The buccal tablet really seems as good to me as an intravenous infusion. This is in my own experience the most effective way to treat therapy-resistant patients with severe recurring angina pectoris. In these patients the withdrawal of intravenous nitroglycerin is not without problems. Despite oral application of large doses of isosorbide dinitrate (120 mg/day) the incidence of anginal attacks reincreases. In this special situation the application of buccal nitroglycerin seems to have advantages; however, clinical experience is not accumulated.

Some more questions remain open when nitroglycerin is given *orally*. But this may take the same history as isosorbide dinitrate. As shown in the past the first-pass effect of isosorbide dinitrate can be overcome by an increase of the dose. Formerly we used 5 mg, today we use up to 80 mg as a single dose. In the same way the oral dose of nitroglycerin had to be increased from 2.6 to 10, 20 mg or more to get reasonable effects and sufficient blood levels. There are studies which show that the bioavailability of the oral form is good and the duration of action is about 6 h. Pulmonary arterial pressure is reduced during the same course of time. The dose-response relationship demonstrates the importance of large doses. Clinical experience with this drug is promising but further studies are needed.

W.-D. Bussmann, MD, Professor of Medicine, Center of Internal Medicine, Department of Cardiology, University Clinic of the Johann Wolfgang Goethe University, D-6000 Frankfurt a.M. (FRG)

Subject Index

Aminophylline 62
airway resistance 61
hemodynamics 57
pulmonary artery pressure 59
Angina pectoris attack
duration 140
frequency 138
onset 138
treatment 141

Bioavailability 35
Body plethysmography 57
Buccal Synchron nitroglycerin (BGTN; buccal Synchron GTN) 71, 75, 118, 144, 166, 177, 203
acceptance by patient 168, 181
changes of taste 182
during drinking 151, 168, 182
during eating 151, 168, 181, 182
during sleeping 181
during speaking 151, 168, 182
acute action 104, 106
acute prophylactic effect 132
anti-anginal effect 173
buccal mucosa (erythema) 157, 180, 182
cardiac output 104
clinical chemistry 94
cold exposure interval 132
dissolution
dosage scheme 177
mean time 180
rate 156
time 151, 180
dizziness 168
dosage 167
adjustment 182
concomitant administration of propranolol 167
scheme 181
without propranolol 167
dose titration 153, 156
duration of action 151, 211
duration of exercise 168
ergometric load 85, 145, 167
angina pectoris 85
blood pressure 87
changes in ECG 85
duration of exercise 85, 145, 147
exercise tolerance 85
exhaustion 85
heart rate 87
oxygen consumption 94
reproducibility 145
ST segment 147
training effect 154
erythema (buccal mucosa) 157, 180, 182
flushing 168
frequency of attacks 156
headache 112, 156, 157, 168, 203
heart rate 104, 117
hemodynamics 211
influencing factors 22

chewing 22
liquids 22
mouth dryness 22
salivary flow 22
initial dose 183
left ventricular end-diastolic pressure 112
long-term protection 133
maximal hemodynamic effect 151
maximum of effect 121, 151
minimum initial dose 152
mode of application 213
onset of action 212
orthostatic hypotension 168
patient compliance 213
pharmacokinetics 210
pulmonary artery pressure 75, 102
at rest 75, 108
under load 78, 80, 108–112, 114
release curves 22
side effects 89, 94, 112, 151, 182
burning sensation 151, 180, 182
changes in ECG 112
headache 94, 151, 180, 182
hypotension 97
orthostatic hypotension 151
taste 180
tickling 180, 182
tingling sensation 151
vertigo 182
ST segment 82, 84
^{99m}Tc scintigraphy 18, 20

Cold exposure 123, 129, 132, 133
casuistics 127
duration of attack 132
duration of exposure 132, 142
frequency of attack 132
heart rate 129
hemodynamic parameters 123
long-term ECG 127
phenomenology 129
protective mechanisms 123
enhanced metabolism 123
peripheral vasoconstriction 123
ST segment 131
temperature exposure 127
Cold-induced angina pectoris 123, 127, 135
coronary spasm 135
pathogenesis 135
protective reflex mechanism 135
Controlled release formulations
compliance 17
matrix system 17
release mechanism 17
release rate 24
pellet system 17
release mechanism 17
release rate 24
Crescendo-angina 11

Development of tolerance, *see* Nitrates
Diazoxide 50
sodium and water retention 50
Digital plethysmography 35
areas under curve (AUC) 37
diastolic amplitude 37
methodology 35
systolic amplitude 37
variability 43
Dose titration, *see* Titration

First pass effect 5
Frequency-induced angina pectoris 98
duration of attack 99
end-diastolic pressure, left ventricle 98
pacing-induced heart rate 98
systolic pressure, left ventricle 98

History of nitrate administration 4
Hydralazine, sodium and water retention 50

Instable (unstable) angina pectoris 9
coronary vasospasm 9
nitrates 10
Isosorbide dinitrate (ISDN)
cardiac output 186
development of tolerance 1
dose-response relationship 1
headache 203
heart rate 186
left ventricular stroke work index 186
pulmonary artery pressure 186
pulmonary wedge pressure 186
right atrial pressure 186

Isosorbide dinitrate *(cont.)*
stroke volume 186
systemic arterial pressure 186
Isosorbide-5'-mononitrate (IS-5-mononitrate) 1, 203
headache 203

Left ventricular ejection time, *see* Systolic time intervals

Minoxidil, sodium and water retention 50

Nitrates
ascites 56
dosage 6, 10
edema 56
first pass effect 24
heart failure (congestive) 6, 8, 10, 54, 56
hyperaldosteronism 54
indications 7
cardiac 8
non-cardiac 8
metabolism 5
mode of application (delivery systems) 10, 11
disk 10
nasal spray 10
ointment 10
myocardial infarction 8, 9
area 9
pain 9
myocardial perfusion 9
Q wave 9
renal blood flow 54
sensitivity 7
sodium and water retention 54
tolerance 7, 14
Nitroglycerin
adsorptivity to plastic 26
high-density polyethylene 33
non-adsorbing infusing instruments 33
plastic bags and tubes 33
polyvinylchloride 33
concentration at the site of action 32
erythrocyte concentration
erythrocyte/plasma quotient in humans 30
erythrocyte/plasma quotient in rats 30
instability 26
tissue concentration 32, 33
volatility 26
Nitroglycerin determination, *see* Plasma nitroglycerin concentration
Nitroglycerin plasma concentration 45
intersubject variability 47
intrasubject variability 48
nitroreductase 44, 48
hepatic 44
organic 48
sensitivity of concentration test 47

Oral Synchron nitroglycerin 184, 187, 211–213
antianginal effect 212
bioavailability 213
blood pressure 186
cardiac output 186
clinical chemistry 200
dosage 211, 212
dose dependency 201
dose increase 201, 203, 213
dose-response relationship 208, 211, 213
duration of action 206, 211, 213
equipotency with ISDN 192, 209
ergometric load 187, 196
blood pressure 196
cardiac arrhythmias 196
cardiac output 188
duration of exercise 196
exercise tolerance 196
heart rate 196
pulmonary artery pressure 187
pulmonary wedge pressure 187
ST segment 196
first-pass effect 193
frequency of attacks 195, 212
gastrointestinal passage 19
general state of health 202
heart rate 186
left ventricular stroke work index 186
maximum of effect 191
plasma concentration 188, 190
pulmonary artery pressure 186, 213

pulmonary wedge pressure 186
renin-angiotensin-aldosterone system 210
right atrial pressure 186
side effects 191, 197, 212
headache 191, 197, 202, 203, 212
heartburn 197
nausea 197
ST segment 205
stroke volume 186
subjective feeling 200
cardiovascular system 200
Freiburg list of complaints 200
gastrointestinal tract 200
general health 200
sum of complaints 200
^{99m}Tc scintigraphy 18, 20, 21
titration 195, 201, 203, 211

PEP, PEP/LVET, *see* Systolic time intervals
Plasma nitroglycerin concentration
half-life
blood vessels 32
plasma 32
method of determination 26–28
atmospheric nitroglycerin 27
blank blood sample 29
chromatography 28, 29
internal standard 28
natural nitro bodies 33
pretreatment with silver nitrate 33
reproducibility 28
silanization of glass instruments 27, 33
standard samples 28, 29
pharmacokinetics 29
distribution volume 29
half-life 29
interindividual deviations 29
intersubject variability 29
plasma clearance 29
plasma clearance
in arterial vessels 31
in the vein 31
site of blood collection 31
Plasma-renin concentration (PRC) 51, 52
Plasma-vasopressin concentration 51, 52
Prazosine, sodium and water retention 50
Pulmonary artery pressure 59
respiratory-dependent oscillations 59
QS_2, *see* Systolic time intervals

Sublingual nitroglycerin 57, 76, 119, 147, 165, 213, 240
acute effect 104, 106
airway resistance 61, 62
cardiac output 104
clinical chemistry 94
duration of action 121, 213
duration of exercise 147
ergometric load 85
blood pressure 85
changes in ECG 85
duration of exercise 85
exercise tolerance 85
exhaustion 85
heart rate 87
oxygen consumption 94
heart rate 104
hemodynamics 57, 61, 62
lung function 62
onset of action 213
peripheral resistance 62
plasma concentration 213
pulmonary artery pressure 59, 75, 108
at rest 75, 108
under load 78, 80, 108, 110, 111, 114
side effects 94
changes in ECG 112
headache 94, 112
ST segment 82
^{99m}Tc scintigraphy 18, 20, 21
Synchron controlled release technology 210
Systolic time intervals 117
left ventricular ejection time (LVET) 119
pre-ejection period (PEP) 118
ratio PEP/LVET 119
total electromechanic systole (QS_2) 117

Titration 155–157, 166, 167, 176
heart rate 144, 145, 167, 176
individual titrated dose 170
initial dose 176
optimum dosage 176
orthostatic hypotension 176

Titration *(cont.)*
  period until onset of hemodynamic effects 170
  resting period 176
  subjective symptoms 167
  systolic blood pressure 145, 167, 176
Tolerance, *see* Nitrates

Vasodilators
  arterial vessels 49
  renin-angiotensin-aldosterone system 49
  sodium and water retention 49
  vasopressin secretion 49
  venous low pressure system 49
Von Euler-Liljestrand mechanism 62